*Prescription For A
Healthy Life*

Prescription For A Healthy Life

Mack Rafeal

Noble Publishing

Contents

INDEX **1**

Chapter 1 **3**

Chapter 2 **19**

Chapter 3 **36**

Chapter 4 **55**

Chapter 5 **70**

Chapter 6 **87**

Chapter 7 **104**

Chapter 8 **119**

Chapter 9 **138**

INDEX

Chapter 1: Introduction
1.1 Opening with the importance of health and well-being
1.2 Defining the purpose of the book: providing a comprehensive guide to a healthy life
1.3 Emphasizing the mind-body connection

Chapter 2: Understanding Health
2.1 Exploring the holistic concept of health
2.2 Discussing the physical, mental, and emotional components of well-being
2.3 Addressing common misconceptions about health

Chapter 3: Nutrition as Medicine
3.1 Highlighting the significance of a balanced diet
3.2 Discussing the role of macronutrients and micronutrients
3.3 Providing practical tips for healthy eating and meal planning

Chapter 4: The Power of Exercise
4.1 Exploring the benefits of regular physical activity
4.2 Discussing different types of exercises for various fitness levels
4.3 Providing a simple exercise routine for readers to follow

Chapter 5: Mental Health Matters
5.1 Addressing the importance of mental well-being
5.2 Discussing stress management techniques
5.3 Exploring mindfulness and meditation practices

Chapter 6: Sleep for Vitality
6.1 Highlighting the importance of quality sleep

6.2 Discussing common sleep disorders and their solutions
6.3 Providing tips for improving sleep hygiene

Chapter 7: Building Healthy Habits
7.1 Discussing the science of habit formation
7.2 Providing practical advice on building and sustaining healthy habits
7.3 Addressing common obstacles and how to overcome them

Chapter 8: Social Connections
8.1 Emphasizing the role of social relationships in health
8.2 Discussing the impact of loneliness and isolation
8.3 Providing strategies for building and maintaining meaningful connections

Chapter 9: Creating Your Personal Health Plan
9.1 Summarizing key takeaways from the previous chapters
9.2 Guiding readers in creating their personalized health plan
9.3 Encouraging ongoing self-reflection and adjustments to maintain a healthy lifestyle

Chapter 1

Introduction

In the mind boggling embroidery of human life, the quest for a solid life is a central string that winds through the texture of our day to day encounters. As we explore the intricacies of innovation, with its high speed rhythms and steadily developing difficulties, the significance of keeping a condition of physical, mental, and profound prosperity has never been more obvious. The mission for a sound life isn't only a transient pattern or a passing trend; rather, it remains as a persevering through yearning implanted in the shared perspective of mankind.

At its center, a solution for a sound life incorporates a comprehensive methodology that rises above the simple shortfall of sickness. It embraces that genuine wellbeing is an agreeable harmony of body, brain, and soul — a sensitive equilibrium that requires intentional and cognizant endeavors. As we dig into the complex components of what comprises a solid life, it becomes obvious that the solution is certainly not a one-size-fits-all cure yet a customized, developing story that adjusts to the consistently changing scenes of our lives.

The groundwork of a solid life lies in the affirmation of the cooperative connection among physical and mental prosperity. Our bodies, unpredictable wonders of organic designing, request mindful consideration and sustaining. From the food we ingest to the rest we enjoy, the actual element of wellbeing unfurls as a material whereupon our everyday decisions paint the image of our general prosperity. The meaning of normal activity, legitimate sustenance, and adequate rest resonates through the passages of clinical insight, shaping the foundation of a proactive remedy for a flourishing presence.

All the while, the scene of psychological wellness arises as a similarly fundamental territory, unpredictably joined with our actual state. In a period set apart by unremitting improvements and a steadily speeding up pace, the safeguarding of mental prosperity requests deliberate practices. Care, stress the executives, and the development of positive idea designs stand as points of support supporting the building of psychological wellness. The remedy for a sound life, consequently, requires a comprehensive coordination of physical and mental prosperity — a consistent dance between the mortal and the cerebral.

However, the forms of a sound life reach out past the individual, reverberating in the aggregate spaces we occupy. Cultural determinants, ecological variables, and the many-sided interaction of networks add to the more extensive material of wellbeing. Tending to wellbeing differences, cultivating inclusivity, and supporting for natural maintainability arise as goals in the all encompassing remedy for a flourishing worldwide local area. The strength of people is inseparably connected to the wellbeing of the networks they occupy, making a harmonious relationship that highlights the interconnectedness of our common human experience.

As we explore the maze of decisions that characterize our regular routines, the significance of preventive consideration arises as a core value in the solution for a solid life. Proactive measures, like routine screenings, immunizations, and wellbeing schooling, act as cornerstones in the curve of prosperity. The shift from responsive to preventive medical services means a paradigmatic development — one that perceives the force of information, early mediation, and the development of wellbeing proficiency in guiding the course of individual and aggregate wellbeing directions.

Besides, the solution for a solid life isn't bound to the domain of the physical and the outer. The inner scenes of feelings, values, and reason contribute essentially to the general embroidery of prosperity. The capacity to understand people on a profound level, the capacity to explore and figure out one's own feelings and those of others, turns into a compass directing people through the recurring patterns of life. Developing significant associations, cultivating a feeling of direction, and adjusting one's activities to profoundly held values become necessary features of the remedy, rising above the limits of the human to contact the spirit.

Chasing a solid life, the job of medical care frameworks and strategies poses a potential threat not too far off. Open and evenhanded medical care turns into a key part in the acknowledgment of the solution for all. The crossing point of general wellbeing drives, innovative headways, and the human dash of sympathetic consideration frames an embroidery of medical care that stretches out a long ways past the bounds of clinical settings. A vigorous medical care framework is one that tends to disease as well as proactively advances wellbeing, including the different requirements of people and networks.

Innovation, a characterizing force in the contemporary scene, expects an essential job in the solution for a solid life. From telemedicine and wearable wellbeing gadgets to man-made brainpower driven diagnostics, the joining of innovation into medical care proclaims another period of customized, open, and proficient arrangements. The cooperative energy between human touch and mechanical development makes a scene where the remedy for a solid life isn't just educated by information yet additionally improved by the sympathetic subtleties of human consideration.

In the midst of the heap components that comprise a solid life, the idea of versatility arises as a core value. Life, by its actual nature, unfurls in capricious ways, introducing difficulties and afflictions that test the texture of our prosperity. The solution for a solid life, thusly, incorporates the development of strength — the ability to return quickly from mishaps, adjust to change, and explore the vulnerabilities of presence. Flexibility turns into a powerful power, forming the story of our lives and injecting it with the solidarity to weather conditions storms and arise on the opposite side, more grounded and more dynamic.

In the mosaic of a solid life, the significance of taking care of oneself arises as a repetitive theme. Taking care of oneself isn't an extravagance held for snapshots of relaxation however a fundamental practice woven into the texture of day to day existence. It envelops the specialty of paying attention to one's body, perceiving the signs of weakness or stress, and answering with sympathy. The remedy for a sound life welcomes people to become dynamic stewards of their prosperity, embracing taking care of oneself as an extraordinary practice that transmits outward, impacting individual wellbeing as well as the more extensive circles of connections, work, and local area.

Training, as an impetus for strengthening and illumination, expects a focal job in the solution for a sound life. Wellbeing proficiency, enveloping a profound comprehension of one's body, mind, and the more extensive determinants of wellbeing, turns into a foundation in the development of a proactive and informed way to deal with prosperity. The remedy reaches out past proper instruction to embrace a consistent excursion of learning — an investigation of the steadily developing scene of wellbeing information that enables people to settle on informed decisions and supporter for their own prosperity.

In the story of a solid life, the elements of euphoria, imagination, and reason arise as fundamental strings that add lavishness and profundity to the embroidery. Euphoria, as a condition of being that rises above flitting bliss, turns into a compass directing people towards exercises and connections that bring satisfaction. Innovativeness, whether communicated through human expression, development, or critical thinking, turns into a unique power that jazzes up the soul and adds to a feeling of imperativeness. Reason, the arrangement of one's activities with a higher calling or mission, turns into a north star that gives guidance and importance to the excursion of life.

All in all, the remedy for a solid life unfurls as a unique story, enveloping the exchange of physical, mental, profound, and cultural aspects. It is an embroidery woven with the strings of preventive consideration, strength, taking care of oneself, and the extraordinary force of training. In the mosaic of wellbeing, innovation and medical care frameworks join with the human touch, making a scene where development and empathy blend for the prosperity of people and networks. As we explore the maze of decisions, the remedy for a solid life welcomes us to be dynamic members in the continuous discourse with our bodies, minds, and our general surroundings — an exchange that shapes the story of a daily existence lived in energetic wellbeing and reason.

1.1 Opening with the importance of health and well-being

In the terrific woven artwork of life, wellbeing and prosperity stand as central strings, winding through the actual pith of our reality. As we cross the multifaceted pathways of our regular routines, the meaning of keeping a condition of ideal wellbeing turns out to be progressively evident. Wellbeing isn't just the shortfall of sickness; a powerful state includes actual essentialness, mental flexibility, and profound balance. The quest for prosperity is a widespread desire that rises above social, geographic, and financial limits, reverberating as a consistent idea that ties every one of us.

At the core of the human experience lies the obvious truth that our prosperity is personally interlaced with the nature of our lives. A solid body gives the material whereupon the shades of our encounters are painted. At the point when our actual wellbeing is hearty, we are supplied with the energy and essentialness to draw in with the world, seek after our interests, and fabricate significant associations. It turns into the very establishment whereupon we develop the structure of our lives — a strong base that permits us to go after the levels of our desires.

Mental prosperity, a feature frequently eclipsed by the conspicuousness of actual wellbeing, is similarly crucial in forming the shapes of a satisfied life. The brain, a complicated snare of considerations, feelings, and discernments, assumes a focal part in our everyday encounters. A solid brain isn't just described by the shortfall of psychological instability yet in addition by the presence of strength, the ability to understand people on a profound level, and an ability to explore the intricacies of life. It is the focal point through which we decipher the world, impacting our perspectives, decisions, and communications with others.

Close to home prosperity, frequently viewed as the spirit's appearance in the waters of our cognizance, adds profundity and subtlety to the material of our lives. The capacity to figure out, express, and deal with our feelings is a sign of the ability to understand individuals on a deeper level — an expertise that adds to the lavishness of our connections and the general personal satisfaction. Close to home prosperity includes perceiving and handling our own feelings as well as identifying with the sensations of others, encouraging associations that are bona fide and satisfying.

In the mosaic of prosperity, the cultural and ecological aspects structure vital bits of the riddle. The people group we possess, the financial designs that shape our chances, and the natural circumstances that encompass every one of us assume critical parts in deciding our wellbeing and prosperity. Perceiving the interconnectedness of individual and aggregate wellbeing highlights the significance of resolving foundational issues, upholding for civil rights, and cultivating conditions that advance the prospering of all.

The quest for wellbeing and prosperity is definitely not a static undertaking yet a continuous excursion — a powerful story that unfurls through our decisions, the propensities we develop, and the viewpoints we embrace. An excursion requires a comprehensive methodology, recognizing the complex interaction between physical, mental, and close to home aspects. The significance of taking on a proactive position in defending our wellbeing couldn't possibly be more significant, as preventive measures and deliberate decisions prepare for a day to day existence portrayed by essentialness, versatility, and satisfaction.

In the contemporary scene, the speed of life frequently appears to speed up, and the requests on our time and consideration can overpower. Amidst these difficulties, the idea of preventive consideration arises as a core value in the solution for a sound life. Instead of trusting that ailment will show, preventive consideration includes proactive measures that thwart potential medical problems. Routine wellbeing screenings, inoculations, and way of life decisions that focus on prosperity add to a story of wellbeing that isn't just responsive yet expectant.

The reconciliation of innovation into the domain of medical care proclaims another period of conceivable outcomes chasing after wellbeing and prosperity. Telemedicine, wearable wellbeing gadgets, and man-made reasoning driven diagnostics are among the advancements that enable people to assume responsibility for their wellbeing in remarkable ways. The marriage of human touch with innovative progressions makes a scene where customized, open, and productive medical care arrangements join, upgrading the general insight of prosperity.

Schooling arises as a strong impetus in the excursion towards wellbeing and prosperity. Wellbeing proficiency, the capacity to comprehend and explore data around one's wellbeing, turns into a foundation in settling on informed choices.

The significance of encouraging wellbeing proficiency stretches out past conventional schooling to envelop a consistent course of learning — one that furnishes people with the information and abilities to advocate for their prosperity and effectively take part in molding the direction of their wellbeing.

The scene of prosperity likewise unfurls inside the domains of happiness, imagination, and reason. Euphoria, as a condition of being that rises above transient joy, turns into a directing power that leads people towards exercises and connections that bring certifiable satisfaction. Imagination, communicated through human expression, development, and critical thinking, adds energy and imperativeness to life. Reason, the arrangement of one's activities with a higher calling or mission, turns into a compass that gives guidance and importance to the excursion of prosperity.

Taking care of oneself arises as a fundamental practice in the solution for wellbeing and prosperity. It's anything but a childish extravagance yet a central part of keeping up with equilibrium and strength notwithstanding life's difficulties. Taking care of oneself includes tuning into one's own requirements, perceiving indications of weariness or stress, and answering with sympathy and deliberateness. A long way from being an extravagance, taking care of oneself is a groundbreaking practice that swells outward, emphatically impacting connections, work, and the more extensive circles of life.

Versatility, the capacity to quickly return from mishaps and adjust to change, turns into a unique power in the story of prosperity. Life, by its actual nature, unfurls in eccentric ways, introducing difficulties and afflictions. Developing flexibility includes enduring tempests as well as arising on the opposite side with newly discovered strength and shrewdness. A quality changes misfortunes into valuable open doors for development and shapes the story of prosperity with an unflinching soul.

Chasing after wellbeing and prosperity, the job of medical care frameworks and approaches can't be disregarded. Open and fair medical services turns into a key part in the acknowledgment of the remedy for all. The convergence of general wellbeing drives, mechanical progressions, and sympathetic consideration shapes an embroidery of medical services that stretches out past the limits of clinical settings. A strong medical services framework is one that tends to sickness as well as proactively advances wellbeing, perceiving the different necessities of people and networks.

The remedy for wellbeing and prosperity reaches out past individual limits, reverberating in the common spaces we possess. The differences in wellbeing results, the social determinants that shape our chances, and the ecological variables that impact our prosperity highlight the requirement for an aggregate way to deal with wellbeing. Backing for civil rights, the making of comprehensive conditions, and feasible practices add to the more extensive story of wellbeing — an account that perceives the interconnectedness of our common human experience.

As we ponder the significance of wellbeing and prosperity, it becomes clear that the solution for a satisfying and energetic life is certainly not a one-size-fits-all cure. It is a customized, developing story that adjusts to the consistently changing scenes of our lives. It welcomes us to be dynamic members in the continuous exchange with our bodies, minds, and our general surroundings — a discourse that shapes the story of a daily existence lived in energetic wellbeing and reason.

All in all, the significance of wellbeing and prosperity couldn't possibly be more significant in the excellent woven artwork of human life. A basic perspective impacts the nature of our lives, molding our encounters, connections, and in general feeling of satisfaction. The quest for wellbeing and prosperity is a diverse excursion that envelops actual essentialness, mental versatility, profound balance, and cultural concordance. It requires a comprehensive methodology, perceiving the interconnectedness of individual and aggregate prosperity. As we explore the complicated pathways of life, the remedy for wellbeing and prosperity welcomes us to embrace a proactive position, coordinate innovation with empathy, encourage wellbeing proficiency, and develop euphoria, imagination, and reason. It is a unique story, winding through the texture of our lives, directing us towards a condition of prospering and dynamic prosperity.

1.2 Defining the purpose of the book: providing a comprehensive guide to a healthy life

At the center of this scholarly undertaking lies a significant obligation to disentangle the unpredictable embroidery of a solid life. During a time set apart by the tenacious quest for progress, the significance of wellbeing frequently becomes the overwhelming focus as a core value for an everyday routine very much experienced. This book sets out on an excursion to characterize, investigate, and enlighten the complex elements of a sound life, expecting to give a far reaching guide that rises above ordinary limits.

The motivation behind this book is grounded in the acknowledgment that wellbeing is definitely not a simple shortfall of disease yet a powerful state enveloping actual essentialness, mental strength, profound prosperity, and a feeling of direction. It tries to explore the maze of present day presence, offering bits of knowledge, procedures, and astuteness to enable people as they continued looking for comprehensive prosperity. The overall objective is to furnish perusers with a tool stash that reaches out past nonexclusive solutions, fitting exhortation to different ways of life, inclinations, and necessities.

In a world immersed with data, the requirement for an exhaustive manual for a solid life turns out to be progressively articulated. The book tries to distil complex ideas into available information, making the quest for wellbeing and prosperity a receptive and educated attempt for perusers regarding all foundations. Through a union of logical examination, functional exhortation, and immortal insight, it tries to overcome any barrier among hypothesis and work on, directing perusers on a groundbreaking excursion toward a better, really satisfying life.

The underpinning of the extensive aide lies in the acknowledgment that wellbeing is a comprehensive idea, requiring a nuanced comprehension of the interconnected aspects that shape our prosperity. While actual wellbeing fills in as a foundation, the book digs into the frequently disregarded domains of mental and close to home prosperity, cultural variables, and the more extensive setting of ecological impacts. By embracing this comprehensive point of view, the aide plans to offer a guide that considers the full range of variables impacting an individual's wellbeing.

One critical part of the exhaustive aide is the accentuation on preventive consideration — a change in perspective from the receptive methodologies that rule contemporary medical care. Rather than trusting that infirmities will show, the book advocates for proactive measures, engaging perusers to go with decisions that prevent potential medical problems. Through viable tips, proof based suggestions, and experiences into the most recent progressions in preventive medical care, the aide tries to impart an outlook that focuses on long haul prosperity.

Innovation, an unavoidable power in the cutting edge scene, expects an unmistakable job in the far reaching guide. From telemedicine to wearable wellbeing gadgets and man-made reasoning driven diagnostics, innovation gives extraordinary devices to people to screen, comprehend, and upgrade their wellbeing. The aide investigates the convergence of innovation and prosperity, offering a nuanced viewpoint on how these developments can be saddled to upgrade individual wellbeing results while exploring the moral contemplations that emerge in this computerized age.

Training arises as a foundation in the extensive aide, perceiving that educated decisions are urgent chasing a solid life. Wellbeing proficiency, the capacity to comprehend and apply wellbeing data, turns into a point of convergence as the aide urges perusers to effectively draw in with their prosperity. Past the customary homeroom, the aide advocates for a consistent learning approach, engaging people to keep up to date with developing wellbeing information and develop a proactive position in dealing with their wellbeing.

The account unfurls inside the domains of happiness, imagination, and reason — aspects frequently neglected in customary conversations of wellbeing. The aide recognizes that prosperity reaches out past the shortfall of sickness to incorporate a daily existence loaded up with euphoric encounters, imaginative articulation, and a feeling of direction. By investigating these aspects, the far reaching guide looks to reclassify wellbeing as an all encompassing and improving excursion, moving perusers to embrace a daily existence that goes past simple endurance and flourishes chasing satisfaction.

Taking care of oneself, an idea that rises above shallow thoughts of spoiling, is complicatedly woven into the texture of the extensive aide. It underlines that taking care of oneself isn't a guilty pleasure yet a central practice that sustains strength, cultivates balance, and advances generally prosperity.

By offering functional systems and experiences into the groundbreaking force of taking care of oneself, the aide expects to engage perusers to focus on their own wellbeing in the midst of the requests of current life.

Versatility arises as a key subject, recognizing that the excursion to a sound life isn't without its difficulties. Life unfurls in capricious ways, introducing snags and difficulties. The aide highlights the significance of developing strength — the capacity to return from mishaps, adjust to change, and arise more grounded. Through genuine models, mental experiences, and pragmatic tips, the aide gives a guide to perusers to explore the inescapable high points and low points of existence with effortlessness and strength.

There is no such thing as the complete aide in disengagement; it is implanted in the more extensive setting of medical services frameworks and approaches. Open and impartial medical care turns into a basic support point, and the aide advocates for foundational changes that focus on the prosperity, everything being equal. It investigates the convergence of general wellbeing drives, innovative progressions, and sympathetic consideration, imagining a medical care scene that tends to sickness as well as effectively advances wellbeing and preventive measures.

Cultural and ecological aspects likewise highlight unmistakably in the thorough aide. Perceiving that wellbeing is definitely not a singular pursuit however an aggregate undertaking, the aide dives into the social determinants that impact wellbeing results. It advocates for comprehensive conditions, civil rights, and feasible works on, winding around a story that stretches out past private prosperity to embrace the thriving of networks and the planet.

As the aide unfurls, it winds around together different strands of information, encounters, and experiences to make an embroidery that mirrors the intricacy and extravagance of a sound life. It perceives that the quest for prosperity is certainly not a one-size-fits-all undertaking and welcomes perusers to leave on a customized venture that lines up with their exceptional necessities and desires. Through drawing in stories, master interviews, and reasonable activities, the aide expects to be a sidekick on the peruser's way to wellbeing — a wellspring of motivation, information, and strengthening.

All in all, the motivation behind this book is to give an exhaustive manual for a solid life that rises above the limits of customary methodologies. It tries to be a reference point of information and insight, enlightening the different elements of prosperity and engaging perusers to explore the intricacies of current existence with versatility, euphoria, and reason. Grounded in a comprehensive comprehension of wellbeing, the aide welcomes people to become dynamic members in their prosperity, encouraging a proactive mentality that stretches out past the shortfall of disease to embrace a daily existence that twists in the entirety of its aspects.

1.3 Emphasizing the mind-body connection

In the investigation of an extensive manual for a sound life, the entwined connection between the brain and body arises as a focal topic. The brain body association, an idea established in old insight and progressively upheld by current logical figuring out, highlights the significant effect of mental and profound prosperity on actual wellbeing. This story tries to dive into the complexities of this association, underscoring its importance chasing an all encompassing and flourishing life.

At its quintessence, the brain body association mirrors the complex dance between our viewpoints, feelings, and actual prosperity. The affirmation that psychological and profound states can impact physical processes as well as the other way around structures the fundamental rule of this interconnected relationship. Conventional recuperating rehearses, like Ayurveda and Customary Chinese Medication, have long perceived the significance of concordance among brain and body, and contemporary examination keeps on disclosing the physiological components that support this significant association.

One of the critical features of the brain body association is the effect of weight on generally speaking wellbeing. Stress, whether persistent or intense, triggers an outpouring of physiological reactions, delivering chemicals like cortisol and adrenaline. While these reactions are versatile for the time being, ongoing pressure can prompt a large group of medical problems, including cardiovascular issues, compromised insusceptible capability, and incendiary circumstances. Understanding pressure as not exclusively a psychological or close to home peculiarity but rather one with substantial actual repercussions highlights the all encompassing nature of prosperity.

On the other hand, the job of actual wellbeing in molding mental and close to home prosperity is similarly significant. Ordinary activity, for instance, has been displayed to work on actual wellness as well as upgrade mind-set, diminish side effects of uneasiness and sorrow, and add to mental capability. The arrival of endorphins, frequently alluded to as "inspirational" synapses, during actual work embodies the many-sided interchange between substantial development and mental states. This builds up the thought that really focusing on the body is, basically, a type of taking care of oneself for the psyche.

The brain body association reaches out to the domain of insusceptible capability, featuring the impact of mental and close to home variables on the body's capacity to avoid sicknesses. Studies demonstrate that positive feelings, a feeling of direction, and social connectedness can add to a strong safe framework. In actuality, tenacious pessimistic feelings, social disconnection, and ongoing pressure can think twice about capability, making people more helpless to contaminations and sicknesses. This highlights the significant effect that psychological and profound prosperity can have on the body's capacity to keep up with wellbeing.

In the extensive manual for a sound life, supporting the brain body association includes taking on rehearses that advance concordance between these two fundamental parts of human experience. Care, a training established in old pondering practices, has earned respect in contemporary settings for its capacity to upgrade familiarity with the current second and develop a feeling of mental tranquility. Care based intercessions have been displayed to diminish pressure, mitigate side effects of nervousness and discouragement, and add to by and large prosperity.

Mental conduct methods, one more significant device in cultivating the brain body association, include distinguishing and testing pessimistic idea designs that add to pressure and close to home pain. By reshaping mental cycles, people can moderate the effect of weight on both mental and actual wellbeing. These methodologies highlight the pliability of the psyche body association — how deliberate mental practices can apply substantial consequences for physiological prosperity.

The brain body association likewise tracks down articulation in the domain of psychosomatic side effects, where profound or mental elements manifest as actual side effects. Conditions like bad tempered entrail disorder (IBS), strain migraines, and constant torment frequently have establishes in the complicated transaction between mental states and physical processes. Perceiving and addressing the fundamental close to home supporters of these side effects turns into a basic part of all encompassing medical services, recognizing that mending includes keeping an eye on both mental and actual aspects.

Rest, an essential part of generally speaking wellbeing, remains as a powerful illustration of the brain body association. The nature of rest is unpredictably connected to mental prosperity, mental capability, and close to home flexibility. Then again, psychological wellness conditions, like uneasiness and despondency, can fundamentally affect rest designs. The bidirectional idea of this relationship features the requirement for a complete methodology that tends to both rest cleanliness and mental prosperity to enhance this fundamental part of wellbeing.

Nourishment, frequently related fundamentally with actual wellbeing, likewise assumes a urgent part in the brain body association. Arising research demonstrates that the stomach microbiome, a mind boggling environment of microorganisms living in the gastrointestinal system, conveys bidirectionally with the cerebrum. This correspondence organization, known as the stomach mind pivot, impacts temperament, mental capability, and close to home states. An eating routine wealthy in different, supplement thick food varieties contributes not exclusively to actual wellbeing yet in addition to the equilibrium of the stomach microbiome, in this manner affecting mental prosperity.

The brain body association unfurls inside the more extensive setting of the capacity to appreciate people on a profound level — a singular's capacity to perceive, comprehend, and deal with their own feelings, as well as relate to the feelings of others.

The capacity to understand people on a deeper level turns into a vital expertise in exploring the intricacies of connections, cultivating flexibility, and advancing in general prosperity. It includes developing mindfulness, directing feelings really, and encouraging sympathetic associations — an interaction that adds to both mental and actual wellbeing.

The idea of psychoneuroimmunology further highlights the complex exchange between the brain and the safe framework. This interdisciplinary field investigates the manners by which mental variables, like pressure and feelings, impact the anxious and safe frameworks. Understanding the effect of mental and profound states on insusceptible capability gives bits of knowledge into how all encompassing prosperity includes keeping an eye on the brain body association for ideal well-being results.

Care based pressure decrease (MBSR), an organized program created by Dr. Jon Kabat-Zinn, embodies the viable utilization of the psyche body association in medical services. MBSR coordinates care reflection and mindfulness practices to upgrade pressure flexibility and advance generally speaking prosperity. Research on MBSR has shown its adequacy in lessening side effects of uneasiness and misery, further developing rest quality, and in any event, impacting the statement of qualities connected with resistant capability.

With regards to ongoing agony, which frequently has both physical and mental parts, mind-body approaches like mental social treatment (CBT) and care based mediations have shown guarantee in mitigating languishing. By tending to the mental parts of agony and advancing self-viability, these methodologies add to an exhaustive treatment technique that perceives the indivisible idea of mental and actual prosperity.

The brain body association additionally saturates the experience of ongoing ailments, molding the excursion of people confronting conditions like diabetes, cardiovascular illness, or immune system issues. Integrative methodologies that consider the psychological and profound elements of wellbeing become vital parts of all encompassing consideration. The development of flexibility, methods for dealing with hardship or stress, and encouraging groups of people all add to a more thorough way to deal with overseeing ongoing circumstances.

As people explore the intricacies of present day life, the brain body association turns into a core value in the solution for a sound and satisfying presence. Rehearses that advance mental and close to home prosperity, like reflection, yoga, and expressive expressions, offer pathways to develop this association. These practices add to pressure decrease as well as encourage a more profound comprehension of the mind boggling transaction among mental and actual states.

The brain body association is especially piercing with regards to emotional well-being, where conditions like sorrow, uneasiness, and post-horrible pressure problem (PTSD) are progressively perceived as complicated interactions of natural, mental, and social variables.

Integrative methodologies that envelop psychotherapy, drug when vital, and way of life mediations become fundamental in tending to the diverse idea of emotional wellness challenges.

Chasing an exhaustive manual for a solid life, the accentuation on the psyche body association fills in as a compass that explores people toward a coordinated way to deal with prosperity. It highlights the significance of recognizing the indistinguishable idea of mental and actual wellbeing, perceiving that the brain and body are not disconnected elements but rather fundamental aspects of the human experience. This point of view welcomes people to embrace practices, propensities, and mentalities that add to the thriving of both psyche and body, eventually prompting a more energetic and versatile presence.

All in all, the psyche body association arises as a key part in the story of a thorough manual for a sound life. It highlights the significant relationship of mental and actual prosperity, molding the shapes of our encounters, versatility, and by and large wellbeing. By recognizing and purposefully supporting this association, people can set out on an extraordinary excursion toward all encompassing prosperity — one that perceives the cooperative connection between the psyche.

In the extensive scene of wellbeing and prosperity, the brain body association arises as a basic and mind boggling embroidery that winds around together the domains of mental and actual states. This exchange, well established in old insight and progressively validated by logical request, highlights the significant impact that our contemplations, feelings, and mental prosperity employ over our actual wellbeing, as well as the other way around. This story leaves on an extensive investigation of the brain body association, unwinding its subtleties, importance, and suggestions for a comprehensive and flourishing life.

At its center, the brain body association encapsulates the significant interconnectedness of mental and actual prosperity. It is a powerful relationship where considerations, feelings, and perspectives impact physiological cycles, and substantial states equally shape mental and close to home encounters. This cooperative dance between the psyche and body is definitely not a simple philosophical idea however a substantial and dynamic power that assumes a significant part in forming our general wellbeing and personal satisfaction.

Antiquated recuperating customs, like Ayurveda, Customary Chinese Medication, and different pensive practices, have long perceived the indistinguishable idea of brain and body. These practices saw wellbeing as an agreeable harmony between mental, profound, and actual aspects — a point of view that cutting edge science is progressively approving. Contemporary examination in fields like psychoneuroimmunology and social medication dives into the mind boggling systems through which mental and profound states impact safe capability, hormonal equilibrium, and generally wellbeing.

One of the focal principles of the psyche body association is the effect of weight on both mental prosperity and actual wellbeing. Stress, whether got from outside pressures or inner contemplations and feelings, sets off a fountain of physiological reactions. The arrival of stress chemicals, like cortisol and adrenaline, readies the body for a 'instinctive' reaction. While versatile in intense circumstances, constant pressure can prompt a scope of medical problems, including cardiovascular issues, compromised safe capability, and provocative circumstances. This perplexing transaction features the need to see pressure as something beyond a psychological or close to home peculiarity yet as a foundational impact on by and large prosperity.

Understanding pressure inside the setting of the brain body association underlines the significance of all encompassing ways to deal with pressure the executives. Care based pressure decrease (MBSR), for example, incorporates care reflection and mindfulness practices to develop a non-critical consciousness of the current second. Research proposes that MBSR can be viable in lessening pressure, working on profound prosperity, and in any event, impacting physiological markers of wellbeing. This highlights the potential for deliberate mental practices to apply substantial impacts on both mental and actual prosperity.

Additionally, persistent pressure has been connected to conditions like cardiovascular infection, hypertension, and gastrointestinal issues. The brain body association in these examples uncovers the perplexing manners by which mental and profound states add to the turn of events and movement of actual sicknesses. Integrative ways to deal with wellbeing that recognize this association might include pressure decrease strategies, psychotherapy, and way of life alterations to address both the underlying drivers and indications of stress-related conditions.

On the other hand, the positive effect of actual wellbeing rehearses on mental prosperity enlightens the equal idea of the psyche body association. Normal activity, for instance, adds to actual wellness as well as has been displayed to reduce side effects of nervousness and wretchedness. The arrival of endorphins, frequently alluded to as 'feel-great' synapses, during active work represents how substantial developments can impact mental states. This bidirectional relationship highlights that really focusing on the body is intrinsically a type of taking care of oneself for the psyche.

The brain body association expands its impact into the domain of resistant capability, revealing insight into how mental and profound states can adjust the body's capacity to fight off sicknesses. Positive feelings, a feeling of direction, and social connectedness have been related with a fortified insusceptible framework. In actuality, diligent pessimistic feelings, social separation, and persistent pressure can think twice about capability, making people more vulnerable to contaminations and sicknesses. This comprehensive comprehension of the safe framework underscores the significance of mental and profound prosperity in keeping up with generally speaking wellbeing.

Rest, a basic part of prosperity, represents the close connection inside the brain body association. The nature of rest is unpredictably connected to psychological wellness, mental capability, and close to home flexibility. On the other hand, psychological wellness conditions, like uneasiness and despondency, can fundamentally influence rest designs. Tending to rest related issues includes perceiving the corresponding impact between mental prosperity and rest cleanliness, displaying how intercessions focusing on one part of the psyche body association can have flowing consequences for generally wellbeing.

Prescription For A Healthy Life

Nourishment, frequently related essentially with actual wellbeing, likewise assumes a critical part in the brain body association. Arising research in the field of wholesome psychiatry investigates the effect of diet on psychological wellness. The stomach mind hub, a bidirectional correspondence network between the stomach and the cerebrum, represents how the microbiome — microorganisms dwelling in the gastrointestinal system — can impact temperament, mental capability, and close to home states. An eating routine wealthy in different, supplement thick food varieties upholds actual wellbeing as well as sustains the equilibrium of the stomach microbiome, adding to mental prosperity.

The capacity to appreciate people on a profound level, an idea indispensable to the brain body association, epitomizes a singular's capacity to perceive, comprehend, and deal with their own feelings, as well as understand the feelings of others. The capacity to understand people on a deeper level turns into a vital expertise in exploring the intricacies of connections, encouraging flexibility, and advancing generally prosperity. It includes developing mindfulness, directing feelings really, and cultivating sympathetic associations — an interaction that adds to both mental and actual wellbeing.

The brain body association tracks down articulation in psychosomatic side effects, where close to home or mental variables manifest as actual side effects. Conditions like crabby gut disorder (IBS), strain migraines, and persistent agony frequently have establishes in the mind boggling transaction between mental states and normalphysical processes. Perceiving and addressing the fundamental profound supporters of these side effects turns into a basic part of comprehensive medical care, recognizing that mending includes keeping an eye on both mental and actual aspects.

Persistent sicknesses, like diabetes, cardiovascular sickness, or immune system problems, further outline the brain body association with regards to wellbeing. Integrative methodologies that consider the psychological and profound elements of wellbeing become urgent parts of all encompassing consideration. The development of strength, survival methods, and encouraging groups of people all add to a more far reaching way to deal with overseeing persistent circumstances, perceiving that the psyche and body are basic features of the human experience.

Chasing a thorough manual for a solid life, supporting the psyche body association includes taking on rehearses that advance congruity between these two necessary parts of human experience. Care, mental conduct strategies, and other brain body mediations offer pathways to develop this association. These practices add to pressure decrease as well as cultivate a more profound comprehension of the mind boggling interchange among mental and actual states. Coordinating such practices into day to day existence turns into an all encompassing way to deal with prosperity — one that perceives the indistinguishable idea of the psyche and body and enables people to develop a flourishing, incorporated, and satisfying life.

As people explore the intricacies of current life, the psyche body association turns into a core value in the solution for a solid and satisfying presence. Rehearses that advance mental and close to home prosperity, like reflection, yoga, and expressive expressions, offer pathways to develop this association. These practices add to pressure decrease as well as encourage a more profound comprehension of the mind boggling transaction among mental and actual states.

The brain body association is especially powerful with regards to emotional wellbeing, where conditions like sorrow, nervousness, and post-horrendous pressure problem (PTSD) are progressively perceived as intricate interchanges of natural, mental, and social variables. Integrative methodologies that envelop psychotherapy, medicine when important, and way of life mediations become fundamental in tending to the complex idea of psychological well-being difficulties.

Chapter 2

Understanding Health

Understanding wellbeing is a multi-layered try that rises above the simple shortfall of sickness. It envelops an all encompassing viewpoint, recognizing the perplexing exchange of physical, mental, and social prosperity. Chasing a thorough comprehension of wellbeing, one should explore through the maze of organic complexities, mental elements, and cultural impacts that on the whole shape the human experience.

At its center, wellbeing is many times described by the usefulness and equilibrium of the body's physiological frameworks. The mind boggling dance of organs, tissues, and cells organizes an ensemble of life-supporting cycles. From the cadenced thumping of the heart to the multifaceted motioning inside the sensory system, the human body works as a mind boggling and interconnected network. The investigation of life systems and physiology dives into the complexities of this natural wonder, unwinding the secrets of organ frameworks, cell structures, and the biochemical pathways that support life.

However, the idea of wellbeing reaches out past the bounds of actual prosperity. Psychological well-being, a basic part of the general wellbeing range, presents a domain of complexities that explore the scene of feelings, considerations, and ways of behaving. Understanding psychological well-being requires an investigation of the brain's overly complex pathways, diving into the domains of discernment, feeling guideline, and the sensitive equilibrium that describes mental prosperity. The area of brain research unwinds the intricacies of the human psyche, offering bits of knowledge into the elements that add to psychological wellness issues and the techniques for cultivating flexibility and prosperity.

The interconnectedness of physical and emotional well-being turns out to be progressively evident as exploration enlightens the significant effect of mental variables on physiological cycles. The brain body association highlights the unpredictable manners by which close to home states, stress, and mental prosperity impact actual wellbeing results. Ongoing pressure, for example, can appear in an outpouring of physiological reactions, adding to conditions like cardiovascular illnesses, resistant framework dysregulation, and metabolic issues. As the limits between the physical and mental domains obscure, an all encompassing comprehension of wellbeing arises, underlining the requirement for coordinated ways to deal with prosperity.

Cultural elements, as well, apply an imposing impact on wellbeing results. The social determinants of wellbeing, incorporating financial status, training, business, and admittance to medical services, weave an embroidery that essentially shapes people's wellbeing directions. Variations in wellbeing results frequently reflect cultural disparities, highlighting the significance of addressing social determinants to accomplish wellbeing value. The study of disease transmission, the investigation of the dissemination and determinants of wellbeing related states and occasions in populaces, fills in as a pivotal device for unwinding the mind boggling snare of variables that add to wellbeing variations.

General wellbeing drives, directed by epidemiological bits of knowledge, intend to advance populace level wellbeing by tending to modifiable gamble factors, improving medical care access, and encouraging wellbeing advancing conditions. The worldwide wellbeing scene, set apart by both advancement and difficulties, requires cooperative endeavors to handle transferable illnesses, non-transmittable sicknesses, and arising wellbeing dangers. In an interconnected world, where illnesses rise above borders, global collaboration becomes basic to shield worldwide wellbeing security.

The perplexing dance of individual science, mental prosperity, and cultural impacts combines in the medical services framework — a complicated snare of establishments, experts, and mediations intended to advance wellbeing and treat disease. The development of medical care reflects progresses in clinical science as well as the changing elements of cultural assumptions, moral contemplations, and the basic to offset mechanical advancements with sympathetic consideration.

Patient-focused care arises as a change in outlook in medical services, underscoring joint effort between medical care suppliers and patients, esteeming individual inclinations, and recognizing the significance of the patient's voice in navigation. The idea stretches out past the clinical experience, enveloping a more extensive methodology that considers the social determinants of wellbeing and endeavors to address variations in medical care access and results.

The reconciliation of innovation into medical care envoys the two open doors and difficulties. Telemedicine, electronic wellbeing records, and man-made consciousness offer remarkable roads for further developing medical care conveyance, upgrading analytic precision, and customizing therapy plans. In any case, the quick speed of mechanical advancement raises moral contemplations, protection concerns, and inquiries regarding the fair circulation of medical care assets.

Prescription For A Healthy Life

Finding some kind of harmony between saddling the advantages of innovation and safeguarding the human touch in medical services stays a basic test.

Wellbeing training arises as a key part in enabling people to play a functioning job in their prosperity. Wellbeing proficiency, the capacity to get, process, and figure out wellbeing data, turns into a foundation for informed navigation and preventive wellbeing rehearses. Developing wellbeing education outfits people with the instruments to explore the intricacies of the medical care framework, advocate for their wellbeing needs, and pursue decisions that line up with their qualities and inclinations.

The developing scene of medical services conveyance likewise prompts a reexamination of customary models of clinical training. Interdisciplinary joint effort, underscoring the coordination of clinical, nursing, and unified wellbeing callings, becomes basic to address the all encompassing necessities of patients. Group based care models cultivate collaboration among medical services suppliers, advancing far reaching and patient-focused ways to deal with wellbeing.

As the shapes of wellbeing and medical services keep on moving, the basic for exploration and advancement turns out to be progressively obvious. Biomedical exploration tries disentangle the secrets of illnesses, preparing for novel restorative intercessions and preventive methodologies. Translational examination overcomes any barrier between research center disclosures and clinical applications, facilitating the excursion from seat to bedside. The powerful transaction between fundamental science, clinical exploration, and populace wellbeing studies moves the continuum of logical revelation.

Moral contemplations highlight the obligation of established researchers to lead research with uprightness, guaranteeing the government assistance of examination members and the scattering of exact and unprejudiced data.

Bioethics, a field at the crossing point of science, medication, and morals, wrestles with complex inquiries connected with the utilization of arising innovations, the portion of scant assets, and the moral components of medical care direction. As logical progressions push the limits of what is conceivable, moral systems become fundamental advisers for explore the ethical scene of medical care.

The developing idea of wellbeing stretches out past the individual and includes biological aspects. Ecological wellbeing, a discipline that investigates the interconnections between human wellbeing and the climate, reveals insight into the effect of natural variables on infection designs. Environmental change, contamination, and living space annihilation present exceptional difficulties to worldwide wellbeing, requiring purposeful endeavors to moderate natural dangers and advance supportable practices that defend the prosperity of current and people in the future.

The quest for wellbeing value arises as an ethical objective, testing cultural designs that sustain variations in wellbeing results. Value in wellbeing requires not just addressing the social determinants that add to imbalances yet additionally destroying foundational obstructions that limit admittance to medical services, propagate separation, and sabotage the prosperity of minimized networks. The standards of equity and reasonableness become directing signals in the mission to make a medical services scene that focuses on the necessities of the most powerless.

The job of promotion and activism becomes basic to the quest for wellbeing value, enhancing the voices of those whose wellbeing is lopsidedly impacted by fundamental treacheries. Local area commitment, grassroots developments, and strategy support arise as integral assets to drive fundamental change and encourage conditions that advance wellbeing and prosperity for all. The advantageous connection between individual activities, local area elements, and strategy choices highlights the interconnectedness of endeavors to accomplish wellbeing value.

Wellbeing advancement, grounded in the standards of counteraction and strengthening, turns into a foundation for building tough and sound networks. The Ottawa Sanction for Wellbeing Advancement frames key methodologies, underscoring the production of strong conditions, the improvement of individual abilities, the reinforcing of local area activities, the reorientation of wellbeing administrations, and the backing for sound public arrangements. The vision rises above a thin spotlight on medical services mediations, stretching out to the more extensive determinants that shape the circumstances for wellbeing.

As the worldwide scene wrestles with arising wellbeing challenges, the significance of a One Wellbeing approach acquires noticeable quality. One Wellbeing perceives the interconnectedness of human wellbeing, creature wellbeing, and the climate, stressing cooperative endeavors across disciplines to address complex medical problems like zoonotic sicknesses, antimicrobial opposition, and natural dangers.

The synergistic methodology recognizes the relationship of biological systems and highlights the requirement for aggregate activity to protect the wellbeing of the planet and its occupants.

In the domain of irresistible illnesses, the continuous fight against pandemics features the basic for readiness, global collaboration, and the improvement of strong medical care frameworks. The Coronavirus pandemic, a worldwide wellbeing emergency of uncommon scale, highlights the requirement for dexterous reactions, proof based mediations, and impartial dissemination of assets. Examples gained from the pandemic brief a reexamination of general wellbeing systems, emergency the executives, and the basic to construct hearty and versatile medical services frameworks.

Immunization arises as a foundation in the counteraction and control of irresistible illnesses, offering an integral asset to moderate the effect of pandemics. The crossing point of science, general wellbeing, and strategy becomes clear in immunization crusades that expect to accomplish boundless vaccination inclusion.

Nonetheless, antibody aversion, deception, and access boundaries present difficulties to the acknowledgment of worldwide inoculation objectives, accentuating the requirement for exhaustive systems that address the logical angles as well as the sociocultural elements of vaccination.

The field of worldwide wellbeing, at the nexus of global relations, general wellbeing, and philanthropic endeavors, wrestles with the intricacies of tending to wellbeing incongruities on a worldwide scale. Worldwide wellbeing tact turns into a vital instrument in exploring the international scene, encouraging joint effort, and preparing assets to address transnational wellbeing challenges. The moral components of worldwide wellbeing intercessions come to the very front, provoking reflections on power elements, social responsiveness, and the basic to focus on the requirements and voices of the networks impacted by worldwide wellbeing drives.

As the world stands up to the difficulties of the 21st hundred years, the nexus of wellbeing and innovation keeps on advancing, opening new outskirts and moral quandaries. The ascent of accuracy medication, empowered by propels in genomics and customized treatments, holds the commitment of fitting clinical mediations to individual hereditary profiles. Nonetheless, the moral ramifications of hereditary testing, the potential for segregation in light of hereditary data, and the impartial dispersion of state of the art medicines present moral difficulties that request cautious thought.

Man-made consciousness (artificial intelligence) arises as a groundbreaking power in medical care, offering the possibility to change diagnostics, therapy arranging, and medical care conveyance. AI calculations investigate immense datasets to determine bits of knowledge, anticipate illness directions, and upgrade treatment regimens.

While computer based intelligence holds monstrous commitment, moral contemplations encompassing information security, algorithmic predisposition, and the ramifications of depending on mechanized frameworks in medical care require cautious examination to guarantee that mechanical headways line up with human qualities and freedoms.

The idea of wellbeing in the 21st century rises above the customary limits of medication and embraces a more extensive worldview that envelops the interconnected idea of human life. The World Wellbeing Association's meaning of wellbeing as "a condition of complete physical, mental, and social prosperity and not simply the shortfall of illness or sickness" reverberates as a core value in exploring the intricacies of contemporary wellbeing challenges.

Chasing after understanding wellbeing, the joining of assorted points of view becomes fundamental. The stories of patients, networks, medical services suppliers, specialists, and policymakers merge to lay out a far reaching picture of wellbeing that mirrors the lavishness of human encounters. Patient accounts, specifically, offer bits of knowledge into the lived real factors of disease, flexibility, and the extraordinary force of medical care encounters. Paying attention to the voices of those with lived encounters turns into a fundamental component in molding medical services strategies, mediations, and the ethos of empathetic consideration.

The way to a better future requires a pledge to deep rooted learning and a receptiveness to embracing developing ideal models. The powerful idea of wellbeing and the fast speed of logical headways highlight the significance of developing a learning society inside the medical care local area. Persistent expert turn of events, interdisciplinary joint effort, and the incorporation of proof based rehearses become basic to adjust to the developing scene of medical services and to give excellent and patient-focused care.

2.1 Exploring the holistic concept of health

Investigating the comprehensive idea of wellbeing welcomes a nuanced assessment of prosperity that stretches out past ordinary clinical structures. The comprehensive methodology recognizes the interconnectedness of different features — physical, mental, profound, social, and, surprisingly, natural — inside the woven artwork of human life. This point of view on wellbeing rises above the conventional model that barely centers around the shortfall of sickness, encouraging us to consider wellbeing as a powerful balance including different aspects.

At the center of the comprehensive worldview is the acknowledgment that the body isn't just an amount of its parts yet a complicatedly interconnected framework. Conventional clinical models frequently compartmentalize the body, treating individual organs or frameworks in confinement. Be that as it may, the all encompassing perspective values the collaboration of physiological cycles and the effect of one framework on another. This interconnectedness is clear in the significant impact of way of life factors, like eating regimen, exercise, and stress the board, on generally speaking prosperity.

Physiological wellbeing, a basic part of the comprehensive idea, incorporates the multifaceted dance of organic frameworks that support life. From the cadenced thumping of the heart to the perplexing motioning inside the sensory system, the human body works as a wonder of natural designing. Understanding life systems and physiology divulges the secrets of organ frameworks, cell structures, and biochemical pathways, giving a guide to fathom the perplexing components that keep up with equilibrium and homeostasis.

In addition, the transaction among physical and psychological well-being turns out to be progressively obvious as examination digs into the brain body association. Profound states, feelings of anxiety, and mental prosperity apply substantial consequences for physiological cycles, affecting resistant capability, cardiovascular wellbeing, and in general flexibility. This bidirectional relationship highlights the all encompassing nature of wellbeing, underlining the significance of addressing both physical and mental aspects to encourage a condition of ideal prosperity.

Prescription For A Healthy Life

The domain of psychological well-being acquaints a layer of intricacy with the comprehensive idea, diving into the complexities of insight, feeling, and conduct. Brain science, as a discipline, offers experiences into the elements impacting psychological wellness, going from hereditary inclinations to natural stressors. Understanding the human psyche includes investigating the components of cognizance, insight, memory, and the unpredictable transaction of synapses that shape temperament and conduct.

Psychological wellness isn't exclusively the shortfall of mental problems; a continuum ranges from prospering to grieving. Positive brain research, a part of brain research that spotlights on human qualities and prosperity, underlines the development of temperances like appreciation, flexibility, and care. This change in perspective highlights the significance of sustaining positive parts of psychological well-being, rising above a shortfall based model to embrace a more extensive comprehension of prosperity.

The capacity to understand people on a deeper level, an idea inside brain research, further improves the investigation of psychological wellness by featuring the capacity to see, comprehend, and deal with one's own feelings, as well as successfully explore relational elements. Developing capacity to understand people on a profound level adds to the improvement of survival strategies, versatility, and better connections, supporting the comprehensive way to deal with wellbeing that coordinates close to home prosperity into the more extensive embroidery of human thriving.

The social element of wellbeing presents one more layer of intricacy, recognizing the effect of cultural designs, connections, and local area elements on prosperity. Social determinants of wellbeing, including financial status, training, business, and admittance to medical services, weave an embroidery that fundamentally shapes wellbeing directions.

Wellbeing abberations frequently reflect cultural disparities, accentuating the need to address social determinants for genuine wellbeing value.

General wellbeing, as a field, arises as a vital player in unwinding the complicated trap of variables adding to wellbeing variations. The study of disease transmission, a foundation of general wellbeing, researches the circulation and determinants of wellbeing related states and occasions in populaces. This approach rises above individual wellbeing encounters, offering a populace level viewpoint that guides mediations to address modifiable gamble factors, improve medical services access, and establish wellbeing advancing conditions.

Worldwide wellbeing, an expansion of general wellbeing, expands the degree to address wellbeing challenges on a worldwide scale. In an interconnected world, illnesses rise above borders, requiring cooperative endeavors to handle transmittable sicknesses, non-transferable sicknesses, and arising wellbeing dangers. Worldwide collaboration becomes basic to defend worldwide wellbeing security, mirroring the common obligation of the worldwide local area to answer wellbeing challenges all in all.

The medical services framework, as an organization, assumes a urgent part in the all encompassing way to deal with wellbeing. Developing over hundreds of years, medical care reflects propels in clinical science as well as changing cultural assumptions, moral contemplations, and the basic to offset mechanical advancements with sympathetic consideration. Patient-focused care arises as a change in perspective, stressing joint effort between medical services suppliers and patients, esteeming individual inclinations, and recognizing the significance of the patient's voice in direction.

The coordination of innovation into medical care messengers the two amazing open doors and difficulties. Telemedicine, electronic wellbeing records, and man-made brainpower offer exceptional roads for further developing medical services conveyance, improving demonstrative exactness, and customizing therapy plans. Notwithstanding, the fast speed of mechanical development raises moral contemplations, protection concerns, and inquiries regarding the impartial circulation of medical care assets. Finding some kind of harmony between bridling the advantages of innovation and protecting the human touch in medical care stays a basic test.

Wellbeing training turns into a key part in enabling people to play a functioning job in their prosperity. Wellbeing proficiency, the capacity to get, process, and figure out wellbeing data, furnishes people with the instruments to explore the intricacies of the medical services framework, advocate for their wellbeing needs, and settle on decisions that line up with their qualities and inclinations. Developing wellbeing proficiency adds to informed navigation and cultivates a feeling of organization in dealing with one's wellbeing.

The developing scene of medical services conveyance prompts a reconsideration of customary models of clinical training. Interdisciplinary cooperation, stressing the reconciliation of clinical, nursing, and associated wellbeing callings, becomes basic to address the all encompassing necessities of patients. Group based care models encourage cooperative energy among medical services suppliers, advancing extensive and patient-focused ways to deal with wellbeing.

As the shapes of wellbeing and medical services keep on moving, the basic for examination and development turns out to be progressively evident. Biomedical exploration attempts disentangle the secrets of illnesses, preparing for novel helpful mediations and preventive systems. Translational exploration overcomes any issues between research center disclosures and clinical applications, speeding up the excursion from seat to bedside. The unique interaction between fundamental science, clinical exploration, and populace wellbeing studies moves the continuum of logical revelation.

Prescription For A Healthy Life

Moral contemplations highlight the obligation of mainstream researchers to direct research with honesty, guaranteeing the government assistance of examination members and the dispersal of exact and impartial data. Bioethics, a field at the convergence of science, medication, and morals, wrestles with complex inquiries connected with the utilization of arising innovations, the designation of scant assets, and the moral elements of medical services independent direction. As logical progressions push the limits of what is conceivable, moral structures become fundamental advisers for explore the ethical scene of medical care.

The developing idea of wellbeing stretches out past the individual and incorporates environmental aspects. Ecological wellbeing, a discipline that investigates the interconnections between human wellbeing and the climate, reveals insight into the effect of natural variables on illness designs. Environmental change, contamination, and natural surroundings annihilation present remarkable difficulties to worldwide wellbeing, requiring deliberate endeavors to alleviate ecological dangers and advance maintainable practices that protect the prosperity of current and people in the future.

The quest for wellbeing value arises as an ethical goal, testing cultural designs that sustain variations in wellbeing results. Value in wellbeing requires not just addressing the social determinants that add to disparities yet additionally destroying foundational obstructions that limit admittance to medical services, sustain separation, and subvert the prosperity of underestimated networks. The standards of equity and reasonableness become directing reference points in the mission to make a medical services scene that focuses on the necessities of the most helpless.

The job of backing and activism becomes indispensable to the quest for wellbeing value, intensifying the voices of those whose wellbeing is lopsidedly impacted by foundational treacheries.

Local area commitment, grassroots developments, and strategy backing arise as amazing assets to drive foundational change and cultivate conditions that advance wellbeing and prosperity for all. The cooperative connection between individual activities, local area elements, and strategy choices highlights the interconnectedness of endeavors to accomplish wellbeing value.

Wellbeing advancement, grounded in the standards of counteraction and strengthening, turns into a foundation for building versatile and sound networks. The Ottawa Contract for Wellbeing Advancement frames key techniques, underscoring the production of steady conditions, the improvement of individual abilities, the reinforcing of local area activities, the reorientation of wellbeing administrations, and the promotion for solid public strategies. The vision rises above a restricted spotlight on medical services mediations, stretching out to the more extensive determinants that shape the circumstances for wellbeing.

As the worldwide scene wrestles with arising wellbeing challenges, the significance of a One Wellbeing approach acquires noticeable quality. One Wellbeing perceives the interconnectedness of human wellbeing, creature wellbeing, and the climate, stressing cooperative endeavors across disciplines to address complex medical problems like zoonotic infections, antimicrobial opposition, and natural dangers. The synergistic methodology recognizes the relationship of biological systems and highlights the requirement for aggregate activity to protect the soundness of the planet and its occupants.

In the domain of irresistible sicknesses, the continuous fight against pandemics features the basic for readiness, worldwide participation, and the advancement of strong medical care frameworks. The Coronavirus pandemic, a worldwide wellbeing emergency of extraordinary scale, highlights the requirement for coordinated reactions, proof based mediations, and fair dissemination of assets. Examples gained from the pandemic brief a reexamination of general wellbeing procedures, emergency the executives, and the basic to fabricate powerful and versatile medical services frameworks.

Immunization arises as a foundation in the counteraction and control of irresistible sicknesses, offering an incredible asset to moderate the effect of pandemics. The convergence of science, general wellbeing, and strategy becomes apparent in inoculation crusades that expect to accomplish far reaching vaccination inclusion. Nonetheless, antibody aversion, falsehood, and access hindrances present difficulties to the acknowledgment of worldwide inoculation objectives, underlining the requirement for complete systems that address the logical angles as well as the sociocultural components of vaccination.

The field of worldwide wellbeing, at the nexus of worldwide relations, general wellbeing, and compassionate endeavors, wrestles with the intricacies of tending to wellbeing variations on a worldwide scale.

Worldwide wellbeing tact turns into a critical instrument in exploring the international scene, cultivating joint effort, and preparing assets to address transnational wellbeing challenges. The moral elements of worldwide wellbeing mediations come to the front, provoking reflections on power elements, social awareness, and the basic to focus on the necessities and voices of the networks impacted by worldwide wellbeing drives.

As the world stands up to the difficulties of the 21st 100 years, the nexus of wellbeing and innovation keeps on advancing, opening new boondocks and moral quandaries. The ascent of accuracy medication, empowered by propels in genomics and customized treatments, holds the commitment of fitting clinical mediations to individual hereditary profiles. In any case, the moral ramifications of hereditary testing, the potential for separation in view of hereditary data, and the impartial conveyance of state of the art medicines present moral difficulties that request cautious thought.

Man-made consciousness (computer based intelligence) arises as an extraordinary power in medical care, offering the possibility to upset diagnostics, therapy arranging, and medical care conveyance. AI calculations investigate huge datasets to determine bits of knowledge, foresee sickness directions, and upgrade therapy regimens. While man-made intelligence holds colossal commitment, moral contemplations encompassing information security, algorithmic predisposition, and the ramifications of depending on mechanized frameworks in medical care require watchful examination to guarantee that mechanical headways line up with human qualities and freedoms.

The idea of wellbeing in the 21st century rises above the customary limits of medication and embraces a more extensive worldview that envelops the interconnected idea of human life. The World Wellbeing Association's meaning of wellbeing as "a condition of complete physical, mental, and social prosperity and not just the shortfall of sickness or illness" reverberates as a core value in exploring the intricacies of contemporary wellbeing challenges.

Chasing understanding wellbeing, the joining of different viewpoints becomes fundamental. The stories of patients, networks, medical care suppliers, specialists, and policymakers meet to lay out an exhaustive picture of wellbeing that mirrors the wealth of human encounters. Patient stories, specifically, offer bits of knowledge into the lived real factors of disease, versatility, and the extraordinary force of medical services encounters. Paying attention to the voices of those with lived encounters turns into a primary component in molding medical services strategies, mediations, and the ethos of merciful consideration.

The way to a better future requires a guarantee to long lasting learning and a receptiveness to embracing developing standards. The unique idea of wellbeing and the quick speed of logical progressions highlight the significance of developing a learning society inside the medical services local area.

Consistent expert turn of events, interdisciplinary coordinated effort, and the joining of proof based rehearses become basic to adjust to the advancing scene of medical services and to give excellent and patient-focused care.

2.2 Discussing the physical, mental, and emotional components of well-being

Prosperity is a complex build that envelops different features of human life, including the physical, mental, and profound aspects. The transaction between these parts complicatedly winds around the embroidered artwork of a singular's general wellbeing and fulfillment with life. An extensive conversation of prosperity requires an investigation of each aspect, recognizing their interconnectedness and the significant effect they on the whole apply on a singular's personal satisfaction.

The actual part of prosperity is central, addressing the condition of the body and its ideal working. Actual wellbeing isn't only the shortfall of sickness however the presence of hearty physiological cycles that help imperativeness and flexibility. It includes the upkeep of homeostasis, where substantial frameworks work agreeably to support life. Factors like sustenance, exercise, rest, and ordinary clinical check-ups add to actual prosperity, shaping the foundation of a solid and dynamic life.

Sustenance assumes a urgent part in actual wellbeing, giving the fundamental supplements that fuel cell processes, support development, and keep up with organ capability. A fair eating regimen, plentiful in nutrients, minerals, and macronutrients, is principal to supporting the body's metabolic requests. Dietary propensities impact actual wellbeing as well as mental and profound prosperity, as the stomach cerebrum hub highlights the bidirectional correspondence between the stomach related framework and the mind.

Practice is one more vital part of actual prosperity, advancing cardiovascular wellbeing, strong strength, and generally speaking wellness. Ordinary active work upgrades actual wellbeing as well as significantly affects mental and profound prosperity. Practice is related with the arrival of endorphins, synapses that go about as normal temperament lifts, adding to a feeling of prosperity and stress decrease. Also, the advantages of activity stretch out to mental capability, further developing memory, fixation, and generally smartness.

Satisfactory rest is fundamental for physical and mental reclamation, assuming an essential part in the body's maintenance processes and mental working. Lack of sleep can maliciously affect temperament, mental execution, and resistant capability, featuring the interconnectedness of physical and mental prosperity. Focusing on great rest cleanliness is essential for keeping up with ideal wellbeing across various aspects.

Ordinary clinical check-ups and preventive medical services measures add to early recognition and the board of potential medical problems. Evaluating for sicknesses, inoculations, and wellbeing appraisals are indispensable parts of keeping up with actual prosperity. The proactive way to deal with medical services forestalls the improvement of sicknesses as well as cultivates a feeling of control and organization over one's wellbeing, decidedly impacting close to home and mental states.

Changing to the psychological part of prosperity dives into the domain of mental cycles, close to home guideline, and mental thriving. Emotional well-being is a powerful express that includes close to home prosperity, mental capability, and the capacity to adapt to life's difficulties. The area of brain science offers bits of knowledge into the horde factors that impact psychological well-being, including hereditary qualities, climate, valuable encounters, and survival strategies.

Positive brain science, a moderately late change in outlook, stresses the development of qualities and temperances that add to a satisfying life. Martin Seligman, a trailblazer in sure brain research, presented the idea of PERMA, addressing positive feelings, commitment, connections, significance, and achievements — major components that add to generally speaking prosperity. By zeroing in on these points of support, positive brain science tries to upgrade the shortfall of dysfunctional behavior as well as the presence of positive mental states and characteristics.

Prescription For A Healthy Life

The capacity to understand people on a deeper level, an idea inside brain research, assumes a urgent part in mental prosperity by working with the comprehension and the executives of one's feelings and the capacity to really explore social cooperations. People with high capacity to appreciate anyone on a profound level will generally have better psychological well-being results, showing flexibility despite difficulty and keeping up with positive relational connections. The development of the capacity to understand individuals on a profound level adds to close to home prosperity, encouraging mindfulness, compassion, and versatile survival techniques.

The brain body association highlights the unpredictable connection among mental and actual prosperity. Stress, a typical element of current life, can show both mentally and physiologically. Constant pressure is related with unfriendly wellbeing results, including cardiovascular infections, safe framework dysregulation, and psychological well-being problems. Stress the executives strategies, like care, contemplation, and unwinding works out, assume a critical part in moderating the effect of weight on both mental and actual prosperity.

The third aspect, close to home prosperity, incorporates the experience and guideline of feelings. Close to home prosperity isn't about steady bliss however the capacity to explore a scope of feelings successfully, figure out their beginnings, and answer adaptively. Close to home flexibility, a vital part of profound prosperity, empowers people to quickly return from misfortunes, adjust to difficulties, and keep an inspirational perspective on life.

Positive feelings add to profound prosperity, cultivating a feeling of happiness, appreciation, and satisfaction. The expand and-fabricate hypothesis of positive feelings sets that encountering good feelings widens a singular's thought-activity collection and constructs mental assets over the long run. Developing positive feelings, thusly, turns into a pathway to upgrading close to home prosperity and making a cradle against the impeding impacts of pessimistic feelings.

The nature of relational connections essentially impacts close to home prosperity. Social associations, everyday reassurance, and a feeling of having a place add to a good profound state. Forlornness and social separation, then again, are related with unfriendly close to home and psychological well-being results. Constructing and keeping up with significant connections, whether with family, companions, or a local area, is necessary to profound prosperity.

Care and taking care of oneself practices assume a vital part in close to home prosperity, offering devices to control feelings, oversee pressure, and develop a good mentality. Care, established in pondering customs, includes focusing on the current second without judgment. Care based mediations have been displayed to decrease side effects of nervousness and despondency, upgrade close to home guideline, and work on generally speaking profound prosperity.

The combination of physical, mental, and close to home prosperity highlights the all encompassing nature of wellbeing. These aspects don't work in segregation; rather, they impact and shape each other in a unique transaction. For example, normal activity adds to actual wellbeing as well as significantly affects mental and close to home prosperity. Likewise, the mental cycles associated with the ability to understand anyone on a deeper level contribute not exclusively to profound prosperity yet additionally to powerful direction and versatile ways of behaving that decidedly influence actual wellbeing.

The advancement of comprehensive prosperity requires a change in perspective in medical care and cultural mentalities. The World Wellbeing Association's meaning of wellbeing as "a condition of complete physical, mental, and social prosperity and not just the shortfall of illness or sickness" mirrors the yearning for a far reaching comprehension of wellbeing that rises above a reductionist point of view. This all encompassing point of view recognizes the interconnectedness of different aspects and stresses the significance of tending to wellbeing completely.

With regards to all encompassing prosperity, preventive medical care expects a focal job. Preventive medical care centers around keeping up with wellbeing and forestalling the beginning of infections, lining up with the all encompassing way to deal with prosperity. Schooling and mindfulness crusades that advance solid ways of life, emotional well-being proficiency, and close to home versatility add to a culture of counteraction, enabling people to play a functioning job in their prosperity across all aspects.

Working environment health programs, progressively perceived as fundamental parts of all encompassing prosperity, address actual wellbeing as well as mental and profound viewpoints. These projects frequently incorporate drives like wellness exercises, stress the executives studios, and psychological wellness support, perceiving that a comprehensive way to deal with prosperity stretches out past the bounds of clinical mediations.

2.3 Addressing common misconceptions about health

Tending to normal misinterpretations about wellbeing is significant for encouraging exact comprehension and advancing informed independent direction. Deception and legends can sustain unwarranted convictions, impact wellbeing ways of behaving, and even effect medical services results. Scattering these confusions requires a thorough assessment of common fantasies across different wellbeing spaces, from nourishment and exercise to emotional well-being and clinical medicines.

One normal confusion rotates around the thought that a thin body compares to ideal wellbeing, disregarding the multi-layered nature of prosperity. While keeping a solid weight is significant for by and large wellbeing, comparing wellbeing exclusively with body size distorts the mind boggling exchange of variables impacting prosperity. Wellbeing includes physical, mental, and close to home aspects, and people with different body sizes can show brilliant wellbeing markers. Weight file (BMI), frequently utilized as a sole mark of wellbeing, has limits, as it doesn't separate among muscle and fat mass or think about circulation. In this way, understanding wellbeing requires a comprehensive viewpoint that thinks about way of life, hereditary qualities, and by and large prosperity.

Another predominant misinterpretation relates to abstain from food and sustenance, with various craze eats less encouraging convenient solutions and extraordinary outcomes. The thought of a one-size-fits-all way to deal with nourishment distorts the complicated connection between diet, individual necessities, and in general wellbeing. While specific dietary examples might be helpful for explicit people, general cases about "superfoods" or outrageous dietary limitations need logical establishing. A fair and differed diet, wealthy in natural products, vegetables, entire grains, and lean proteins, stays a foundation of good sustenance. Customized sustenance plans, custom-made to individual wellbeing needs and inclinations, add to maintainable and successful dietary practices.

The job of fat in the eating regimen has likewise been dependent upon confusions. The "sans fat" or "low-fat" pattern, common in the late twentieth 100 years, spread the possibility that all dietary fat was negative to wellbeing. Nonetheless, not all fats are made equivalent, and fundamental unsaturated fats assume significant parts in physical processes.

Solid fats, like those tracked down in avocados, nuts, and olive oil, add to cardiovascular wellbeing and are fundamental for supplement retention. Figuring out the qualifications between soaked fats, unsaturated fats, and trans fats permits people to pursue informed decisions that help generally wellbeing.

Practice fantasies add to errors about actual work and its effect on wellbeing. A typical confusion is the conviction that exhausting and tedious exercises are the main compelling method for keeping up with wellness. Truly, the vital lies in consistency and finding pleasant exercises that line up with individual inclinations and capacities. Moderate activity, like energetic strolling, moving, or planting, can yield significant medical advantages, including worked on cardiovascular wellbeing, upgraded state of mind, and better weight the executives. The legend that exercise is fundamentally for weight reduction ignores its horde benefits for emotional well-being, bone thickness, and life span.

The possibility that psychological well-being is altogether different from actual wellbeing is another misguided judgment that has acquired conspicuousness. Mental and actual wellbeing are entwined, affecting and influencing each other in a bidirectional way. Mental prosperity adds to actual wellbeing, and then again, actual wellbeing can influence mental prosperity. The shame encompassing emotional wellness issues frequently comes from this bogus polarity, propagating the idea that psychological wellness concerns are inconsequential to generally speaking prosperity. Advancing emotional well-being includes recognizing its essential job in all encompassing prosperity and cultivating open discussions about emotional well-being difficulties.

Misguided judgments about antibodies and their wellbeing have energized immunization aversion, presenting critical general wellbeing gambles. The legend connecting immunizations to chemical imbalance, sustained by a ruined report, has been exposed by broad examination, and various investigations certify the security and viability of immunizations. Inoculation stays one of the best general wellbeing measures, forestalling the spread of irresistible sicknesses and safeguarding people and networks. Tending to immunization related misguided judgments includes giving exact data, exposing fantasies, and developing confidence in mainstream researchers' agreement on antibody wellbeing.

A pervasive fantasy in the domain of clinical medicines revolves around the conviction that normal cures are intrinsically more secure and more viable than ordinary medications. While regular cures can have helpful advantages, expecting that they are generally protected excuses the likely dangers and connections. Also, the "appeal to nature" false notion, which accepts that normal substances are predominant exclusively on the grounds that they are regular, needs logical premise. Integrative medication, which joins proof based ordinary medication with corresponding and elective methodologies, stresses a reasonable and informed way to deal with medical services.

The idea that emotional well-being drugs are an indication of shortcoming or a path of least resistance is another misinterpretation that adds to the shame encompassing psychological wellness medicines. Psychological well-being meds, including antidepressants and temperament stabilizers, assume critical parts in overseeing psychological well-being conditions, frequently revising compound uneven characters in the cerebrum. They are not alternate routes or substitutes for self-improvement and ways of dealing with stress however important instruments that, when recommended and observed by medical services experts, can fundamentally work on people's personal satisfaction.

Another confusion includes the conviction that the human body would be able "detox" through unambiguous eating regimens, enhancements, or practices. The body has its implicit detoxification frameworks, basically including the liver and kidneys, which normally channel and kill poisons. Cases of detox diets or items frequently need logical help and may try and be unsafe. Remaining hydrated, consuming a decent eating regimen, and taking part in ordinary active work are compelling ways of supporting the body's regular detoxification processes.

The relationship of maturing solely with actual downfall and mental crumbling is a typical misguided judgment that adds to ageism. While maturing is related with specific physiological changes, the conviction that all parts of wellbeing definitely decline with age misrepresents the variety of maturing encounters. Numerous more seasoned grown-ups lead dynamic, satisfying lives and keep up with powerful physical and emotional well-being. Testing age-related generalizations includes perceiving the uniqueness of maturing encounters and advancing positive stories about becoming older.

Sexual wellbeing is one more region where misinterpretations proliferate, frequently established in cultural restrictions and lacking schooling. One fantasy is that sexual wellbeing is exclusively about keeping away from physically sent diseases (STIs) or forestalling undesirable pregnancies. Sexual wellbeing envelops a more extensive range, including correspondence, assent, delight, and profound prosperity. Thorough sexual instruction that tends to both the physical and close to home parts of sexual wellbeing is fundamental for dispersing misinterpretations and advancing informed direction.

An inescapable confusion about skin wellbeing rotates around the conviction that a tan is an indication of good wellbeing. The relationship of tanned skin with allure has powered the notoriety of tanning beds and unnecessary sun openness. Truly, drawn out sun openness, particularly without sufficient assurance, builds the gamble of skin malignant growth, untimely maturing, and other skin conditions. Understanding the significance of sun insurance, including sunscreen use and staying away from unreasonable UV openness, is essential for keeping up with skin wellbeing.

The idea of a "wizardry projectile" or a solitary answer for all wellbeing concerns is an inescapable confusion that ignores the independence of wellbeing needs and the perplexing interchange of elements impacting prosperity. Wellbeing is complex, and successful procedures frequently include customized approaches that think about individual ways of life, hereditary inclinations, and ecological variables. Perceiving the variety of wellbeing encounters and embracing fitted mediations adds to a more exact and nuanced comprehension of prosperity.

Tending to confusions about wellbeing requires a complex methodology that includes schooling, open correspondence, and encouraging decisive reasoning abilities. Medical services experts assume a vital part in scattering legends, giving proof based data, and developing a confiding in relationship with patients. General wellbeing efforts, instructive drives, and media education programs add to making a more educated and wellbeing proficient society.

Taking everything into account, tending to normal confusions about wellbeing is basic for advancing precise comprehension and enabling people to settle on informed conclusions about their prosperity. From nourishment and exercise to psychological well-being and clinical medicines, exposing legends includes embracing a comprehensive viewpoint that considers the perplexing transaction of physical, mental, and close to home aspects. By cultivating wellbeing education, advancing proof based data, and testing winning fantasies, society can move towards a more educated and nuanced comprehension of wellbeing.

Chapter 3

Nutrition as Medicine

Sustenance assumes a significant part in keeping up with in general wellbeing and prosperity. Past its key capability of giving energy, food fills in as an amazing asset that can be saddled to forestall and oversee different medical issue. Lately, there has been a developing acknowledgment of the idea of "sustenance as medication," featuring the significant effect that dietary decisions can have on our wellbeing. This change in outlook underlines the significance of survey food as food as well as a strong remedial specialist that can impact the course of illnesses and advance ideal wellbeing.

At the center of the nourishment as-medication reasoning falsehoods the comprehension that the human body requires an equilibrium of fundamental supplements to ideally work. These supplements, including carbs, proteins, fats, nutrients, and minerals, assume basic parts in different physiological cycles. Appropriate nourishment isn't simply about fulfilling yearning or addressing caloric requirements; it is tied in with providing the body with the right blend of supplements in the right extents to help its complex biochemical and metabolic capabilities.

One of the vital standards of involving sustenance as medication is the acknowledgment of the cozy connection among diet and constant sicknesses. Conditions like cardiovascular illness, diabetes, and stoutness, which have arrived at plague extents all around the world, are firmly connected to dietary examples. The Western eating routine, described by high admission of handled food varieties, immersed fats, and refined sugars, has been ensnared in the ascent of these persistent illnesses. Conversely, embracing a supplement thick, plant-based diet has been related with a lower chance of growing such circumstances.

A critical part of sustenance as medication includes grasping the effect of individual supplements on wellbeing results. For instance, omega-3 unsaturated fats, ordinarily tracked down in greasy fish and flaxseeds, have been displayed to have calming properties and may add to cardiovascular wellbeing. Cell reinforcement rich food sources, for example, products of the soil, assume a significant part in killing free extremists and safeguarding cells from oxidative harm, in this way possibly decreasing the gamble of malignant growth and other constant illnesses.

Past macronutrients and micronutrients, the arising field of nutrigenomics investigates how individual hereditary varieties impact reactions to dietary parts. This customized way to deal with nourishment considers a singular's novel hereditary cosmetics, taking into consideration custom-made dietary suggestions in light of hereditary inclinations. Understanding the interaction among hereditary qualities and sustenance opens up additional opportunities for designated mediations that can advance wellbeing results.

In the domain of preventive medication, nourishment becomes the dominant focal point. Embracing a preventive methodology includes settling on dietary decisions that decrease the gamble of creating sicknesses in any case. This proactive position is especially important with regards to non-transmittable infections, where way of life factors, including diet, assume a critical part. General wellbeing drives advancing smart dieting propensities and way of life changes highlight the capability of sustenance as an essential preventive measure.

The significance of sustenance stretches out past forestalling constant illnesses; it likewise assumes a critical part in overseeing existing medical issue. Clinical sustenance treatment, a remedial methodology that use dietary mediations to treat and oversee illnesses, has acquired noticeable quality in different fields of medical services. Conditions like diabetes, hypertension, and heftiness can frequently be really overseen through designated dietary intercessions, decreasing the dependence on pharmacological medicines.

The complicated connection among sustenance and the safe framework features the immunomodulatory capability of dietary decisions. Sufficient nourishment is fundamental for keeping a strong safe reaction, and lacks in key supplements can think twice about body's capacity to battle off diseases.

Alternately, certain food sources, like those plentiful in nutrients C and D, zinc, and cell reinforcements, can upgrade safe capability and add to better guard against microorganisms.

With regards to psychological wellness, the effect of nourishment is progressively perceived as a significant determinant. The stomach cerebrum pivot, a bidirectional correspondence network between the gastrointestinal parcel and the focal sensory system, highlights the association between what we eat and our psychological prosperity. Arising research recommends that the sythesis of the stomach microbiota, impacted by diet, may assume a part in emotional wellness issues, including uneasiness and misery.

The idea of "food as medication" has profound authentic roots, with old societies perceiving the remedial properties of different food varieties and spices. Conventional frameworks of medication, like Ayurveda and Customary Chinese

Medication, have long accentuated the significance of diet in advancing wellbeing and treating sicknesses. In these old practices, food isn't simply a wellspring of sustenance however an integral asset that can reestablish harmony and congruity inside the body.

As we dig into the subtleties of sustenance as medication, it becomes apparent that dietary decisions go past gathering essential healthful requirements. The advanced eating regimen, described by its comfort and overflow, frequently misses the mark in giving the fundamental supplements expected to ideal wellbeing. The predominance of handled food varieties, high in salt, sugar, and undesirable fats, adds to a worldwide wellbeing emergency set apart by increasing paces of heftiness, diabetes, and cardiovascular illness.

In the mission for better wellbeing through sustenance, the job of entire, negligibly handled food varieties becomes the dominant focal point. Entire grains, organic products, vegetables, nuts, and seeds comprise the groundwork of a wellbeing advancing eating routine. These food varieties give a rich exhibit of supplements, including fiber, nutrients, minerals, and phytochemicals, which all in all add to generally speaking prosperity. The accentuation on plant-based sustenance lines up with a developing group of proof supporting the medical advantages of an overwhelmingly plant-centered diet.

The Mediterranean eating routine, frequently proclaimed for its cardiovascular advantages, epitomizes the standards of sustenance as medication. This dietary example, described by maximum usage of organic products, vegetables, entire grains, and olive oil, has been related with a lower hazard of coronary illness and other persistent circumstances. The incorporation of fish, a wellspring of omega-3 unsaturated fats, further upgrades the calming properties of this eating routine.

Rather than the Mediterranean eating routine, the Western eating routine, common in many created nations, is set apart by extreme admission of red and handled meats, sweet drinks, and exceptionally handled food sources.

This dietary example has been connected to an expanded gamble of weight, diabetes, and cardiovascular sickness. The worldwide shift towards Westernized slims down highlights the pressing requirement for intercessions that advance better dietary patterns and bring issues to light about the effect of dietary decisions on long haul wellbeing.

The coming of nourishing science has achieved a more profound comprehension of the particular components through which dietary elements impact wellbeing. Supplement quality cooperations, epigenetic changes, and the balance of flagging pathways give experiences into the unpredictable manners by which nourishment shapes our physiology at the sub-atomic level. This information shapes the reason for designated wholesome mediations that can be custom fitted to individual necessities and wellbeing objectives.

Prescription For A Healthy Life

As we investigate the helpful capability of nourishment, recognizing the restrictions and difficulties innate in making an interpretation of logical information into viable dietary recommendations is fundamental. The intricacy of human digestion, individual varieties in dietary necessities, and the unique idea of wellbeing and sickness present impressive obstacles. Moreover, the impact of financial elements, social practices, and food openness further convolutes endeavors to execute boundless dietary changes.

The field of wholesome the study of disease transmission assumes a vital part in disentangling the connections among diet and wellbeing results on a populace level. Observational examinations, longitudinal associates, and randomized controlled preliminaries add to the assortment of proof that illuminates dietary rules and general wellbeing proposals. In any case, the intrinsic impediments of observational examination, for example, puzzling factors and review predisposition, highlight the requirement for a careful understanding of study discoveries.

With regards to sustenance as medication, the job of dietary enhancements warrants thought. While entire food varieties ought to in a perfect world be the essential wellspring of supplements, enhancements can be an important assistant in specific circumstances. People with explicit supplement lacks, dietary limitations, or ailments that hinder supplement retention might profit from designated supplementation. In any case, the unpredictable utilization of enhancements without an unmistakable clinical sign conveys possible dangers and may not give similar advantages as getting supplements from entire food varieties.

The connection among sustenance and weight the board is a noticeable part of the nourishment as-medication worldview. The stoutness pestilence, filled by inactive ways of life and unnecessary caloric admission, has significant ramifications for wellbeing. Past the corrective worries related with heftiness, for example, self-perception and cultural insights, the wellbeing chances, including diabetes, cardiovascular illness, and certain diseases, highlight the dire requirement for successful techniques to address and forestall weight.

Chasing weight the board, the idea of "calories in, calories out" works on a perplexing exchange of physiological, mental, and natural elements. While energy balance is a central rule, the nature of calories consumed and their effect on digestion, hormonal guideline, and satiety can't be disregarded. Prohibitive weight control plans that emphasis exclusively on caloric admission might disregard the significance of supplement thickness and generally dietary quality.

The reception of an all encompassing way to deal with sustenance includes perceiving the interconnectedness of different way of life factors. Actual work, rest, stress the board, and social help all add to the general wellbeing condition. The combination of these variables into a complete health system improves the viability of dietary mediations and advances practical way of life changes.

In the domain of pediatric nourishment, the idea of sustenance as medication takes on added importance. The early long periods of life address a basic time of development and improvement, and nourishing decisions during this time can affect wellbeing. Breastfeeding, perceived for interesting organization upholds ideal newborn child improvement, is viewed as a foundation of early sustenance. Presentation of strong food sources and the foundation of smart dieting propensities during youth establish the groundwork for deep rooted wellbeing.

Youth corpulence, a rising concern universally, underlines the requirement for designated intercessions to advance good dieting propensities and dynamic ways of life since early on. The impact of parental ways of behaving, ecological elements, and the food business on youngsters' dietary decisions highlights the diverse idea of the test. School-based sustenance training, strategy changes, and local area drives assume crucial parts in molding the food climate for youngsters and cultivating a culture of wellbeing.

The effect of nourishment on mental capability and cerebrum wellbeing is a developing area of examination. The cerebrum, a profoundly metabolically dynamic organ, depends on a consistent inventory of supplements to help its capabilities. Omega-3 unsaturated fats, tracked down in overflow in greasy fish, pecans, and flaxseeds, have been related with mental advantages. Cell reinforcement rich food sources, like berries and mixed greens, may safeguard the mind from oxidative pressure and age-related decline.

The stomach cerebrum pivot, a bidirectional correspondence pathway between the stomach and the focal sensory system, gives a captivating understanding into the interconnectedness of the stomach related framework and mind capability. Arising research recommends that the stomach microbiota, impacted by diet, may assume a part in emotional well-being problems, including despondency and tension. The potential for dietary mediations to balance the stomach microbiome and influence mental prosperity opens up new roads for tending to psychological wellness challenges.

With regards to maturing, nourishment takes on added importance as a determinant of healthspan - the quantity of years a singular remaining parts sound and dynamic. Age-related changes in digestion, supplement assimilation, and bulk feature the requirement for fitted dietary methodologies to help ideal maturing. Satisfactory protein consumption, micronutrient-rich food varieties, and hydration are pivotal components of a nourishment plan that tends to the novel requirements of more seasoned grown-ups.

The predominance of hunger, a condition portrayed by insufficient or overabundance supplement consumption, stays a worldwide concern, influencing people, everything being equal. Unhealthiness envelops undernutrition, overnutrition, and micronutrient lacks, each introducing unmistakable wellbeing challenges. Tending to unhealthiness requires a diverse methodology that joins restorative mediations with general wellbeing drives pointed toward further developing food security, openness, and schooling.

The convergence of sustenance and social variety highlights the requirement for socially delicate ways to deal with dietary proposals. Social convictions, customs, and dietary practices impact food decisions and dietary patterns, forming the nourishing scene of networks all over the planet. Powerful sustenance intercessions should consider the social setting, recognizing and regarding different points of view on food and wellbeing.

The job of medical care experts in advancing nourishment as medication is significant. Coordinating nourishment instruction into clinical educational programs outfits future medical services suppliers with the information and abilities to integrate dietary mediations into patient consideration. Proceeding with schooling for rehearsing clinicians guarantees that they keep up to date with the most recent examination and rules, enabling them to direct patients towards better dietary decisions.

The coordinated effort between medical services experts, dietitians, and different individuals from the medical care group is fundamental for complete patient consideration. A multidisciplinary approach considers a comprehensive evaluation of a singular's wellbeing, considering clinical history, dietary propensities, and way of life factors. This cooperative model empowers the advancement of customized nourishment designs that line up with the singular's wellbeing objectives and clinical requirements.

The advancing scene of innovation and medical care converges with nourishment, offering inventive answers for customized sustenance. Portable applications, wearable gadgets, and telehealth stages give instruments to people to follow their dietary propensities, screen actual work, and get continuous input. These mechanical progressions work with more noteworthy commitment to wellbeing advancing ways of behaving and overcome any issues between conventional medical care and the regular daily existences of people.

The financial ramifications of the sustenance as-medication worldview are significant. The weight of diet-related infections on medical services frameworks highlights the financial advantages of preventive sustenance intercessions. Putting resources into nourishment instruction, local area projects, and strategy drives that advance smart dieting can yield long haul cost reserve funds by lessening the predominance of persistent infections and their related medical care costs.

The food business' part in forming the dietary scene couldn't possibly be more significant. The accessibility, reasonableness, and promoting of food items impact customer decisions and dietary examples. A shift towards better food choices, straightforward naming, and mindful showcasing rehearses lines up with the objectives of advancing sustenance as medication. Cooperative endeavors between the food business, policymakers, and general wellbeing advocates are fundamental for establishing a climate that upholds invigorating dietary decisions.

3.1 Highlighting the significance of a balanced diet

A fair eating routine is a foundation of generally wellbeing and prosperity, addressing a crucial rule that underlies the body's capacity to ideally work. It envelops the utilization of a different exhibit of supplements in proper extents to meet the body's wholesome necessities. The meaning of a reasonable eating routine couldn't possibly be more significant, as it assumes an essential part in supporting development, keeping up with energy levels, forestalling sicknesses, and advancing life span.

At the core of a decent eating regimen is the idea of balance and assortment. This approach guarantees that the body gets a range of fundamental supplements, including starches, proteins, fats, nutrients, and minerals, in amounts that line up with its prerequisites. Every supplement assumes an extraordinary part in supporting fundamental physiological capabilities, and an irregularity in their admission can prompt dietary lacks or overabundances, with impeding impacts on wellbeing.

Starches, as an essential wellspring of energy, are a vital part of a fair eating routine. Found in food sources like grains, organic products, and vegetables, sugars are separated into glucose, which energizes the body's cells and supports different metabolic cycles. Picking complex starches, like entire grains, guarantees a consistent arrival of energy and manages glucose levels, adding to supported energy over the course of the day.

Proteins, including fundamental amino acids, are critical for the body's development, fix, and upkeep. A decent eating regimen incorporates an assortment of protein sources, like lean meats, poultry, fish, vegetables, and dairy items.

Sufficient protein admission is especially significant for muscle improvement, invulnerable capability, and the union of catalysts and chemicals that direct different physiological cycles.

Fats, frequently denounced yet fundamental for wellbeing, are one more part of a fair eating regimen. Solid fats, including monounsaturated and polyunsaturated fats tracked down in olive oil, avocados, and greasy fish, assume a part in supporting cell structure, engrossing fat-dissolvable nutrients, and keeping up with cerebrum wellbeing. Finding some kind of harmony between various sorts of fats and keeping away from extreme immersed and trans fats is vital to advancing cardiovascular wellbeing.

The incorporation of a range of nutrients and minerals is indispensable to a reasonable eating routine. These micronutrients act as cofactors in enzymatic responses, add to bone wellbeing, support safe capability, and go about as cancer prevention agents that shield cells from oxidative pressure. Organic products, vegetables, nuts, seeds, and entire grains are rich wellsprings of nutrients and minerals, stressing the significance of integrating different these food varieties into everyday dinners.

The meaning of water in keeping a fair eating routine can't be ignored. Hydration is fundamental for various physiological cycles, including processing, supplement retention, and temperature guideline. Water is a sans calorie drink that ought to be the essential decision for extinguishing thirst, and its admission is basic for generally speaking wellbeing and prosperity.

A reasonable eating regimen goes past the simple arrangement of fundamental supplements; it likewise thinks about the nature of food decisions. Entire, negligibly handled food sources are the underpinning of a wellbeing advancing eating regimen. These food varieties, in their regular state, hold their inborn dietary benefit, giving a rich exhibit of nutrients, minerals, fiber, and phytochemicals. Conversely, exceptionally handled food varieties, loaded down with added sugars, undesirable fats, and counterfeit added substances, add to the rising tide of diet-related sicknesses.

The effect of a decent eating routine on development and improvement is especially articulated during basic life stages, like pregnancy and outset. Maternal nourishment assumes a significant part in fetal turn of events, impacting the child's wellbeing both in utero and sometime down the road. Satisfactory admission of supplements like folate, iron, and omega-3 unsaturated fats during pregnancy is related with positive results for both the mother and the kid.

In the early long periods of life, a fair eating routine is fundamental for supporting ideal development and improvement. Bosom milk, thought about the highest quality level for newborn child nourishment, gives a special mix of supplements, antibodies, and bioactive mixtures that advance the baby's wellbeing. As the youngster changes to strong food sources, the presentation of a different scope of supplement rich food varieties lays out smart dieting propensities and establishes the groundwork for long lasting prosperity.

The job of a reasonable eating regimen reaches out into immaturity, a period set apart by fast development and actual turn of events. Supplement necessities increment during this stage, stressing the significance of an eating routine that satisfies the needs of a creating body and supports the foundation of solid way of life propensities. Instructing young people about the meaning of sustenance engages them to settle on informed decisions that add to their general wellbeing and flexibility.

Adulthood brings its own arrangement of difficulties, with occupied plans, business related pressure, and way of life factors that might affect dietary decisions. A decent eating regimen becomes instrumental in dealing with these difficulties, giving the important supplements to support energy levels, support mental capability, and forestall the beginning of constant sicknesses. As people age, the nourishing necessities of the body advance, highlighting the significance of adjusting dietary decisions to meet evolving prerequisites.

The effect of diet on persistent illnesses is a significant point of convergence while thinking about the meaning of a fair eating regimen. Non-transferable sicknesses, including cardiovascular infection, diabetes, and certain tumors, are complicatedly connected to dietary examples. The worldwide predominance of these illnesses features the critical requirement for preventive measures, with sustenance assuming a focal part in relieving risk factors and advancing wellbeing.

Cardiovascular wellbeing, specifically, is unequivocally impacted by dietary decisions. An eating regimen wealthy in natural products, vegetables, entire grains, and lean proteins has been related with a lower chance of coronary illness. On the other hand, eats less carbs high in immersed and trans fats, sodium, and added sugars add to the advancement of hazard factors like hypertension, elevated cholesterol, and weight.

The connection among diet and diabetes is one more convincing delineation of the effect of nourishment on wellbeing results. Type 2 diabetes, frequently connected with way of life factors, including diet and actual work, is a preventable and sensible condition. Taking on a fair eating regimen that controls glucose levels, keeps a sound weight, and advances insulin responsiveness is a foundation of diabetes the executives and counteraction.

Malignant growth counteraction is a complicated and complex undertaking, with diet arising as a modifiable gamble factor. The defensive impacts of specific food sources and dietary examples against explicit malignant growths have been a subject of broad examination. Cell reinforcement rich food sources, cruciferous vegetables, and an eating regimen high in fiber have been related with a lower hazard of specific malignant growths, featuring the capability of sustenance as a preventive system.

Corpulence, a worldwide scourge with significant wellbeing suggestions, highlights the meaning of a reasonable eating routine in weight the executives. The interchange of dietary decisions, active work, and metabolic variables decides body weight and creation. Consumes less calories high in refined sugars, undesirable fats, and handled food sources add to unnecessary calorie consumption, while an absence of active work further worsens the gamble of stoutness.

With regards to emotional well-being, the association among diet and temperament is an arising area of examination. The stomach cerebrum hub, a bidirectional correspondence framework between the stomach and the focal sensory system, features the impact of the stomach microbiota on mental prosperity. Certain supplements, like omega-3 unsaturated fats, B nutrients, and cell reinforcements, assume parts in synapse combination and cerebrum capability, recommending a possible connection among diet and emotional well-being results.

Prescription For A Healthy Life

A fair eating routine likewise has suggestions for resistant capability, especially significant with regards to worldwide wellbeing challenges. Sufficient sustenance is fundamental for keeping a vigorous resistant reaction, and lacks in key supplements can think twice about body's capacity to fight off contaminations. The job of explicit supplements, like L-ascorbic acid, vitamin D, zinc, and probiotics, in supporting safe capability is an area of continuous exploration.

The monetary ramifications of a reasonable eating routine stretch out past individual wellbeing to more extensive cultural and medical care contemplations. The weight of diet-related illnesses on medical services frameworks, efficiency misfortunes, and the related financial costs feature the potential for practical preventive estimates through nourishment mediations. Putting resources into general wellbeing drives, nourishment schooling, and strategies that advance good food conditions can yield long haul monetary advantages.

Instructive drives pointed toward bringing issues to light about the meaning of a decent eating routine are vital for engaging people to pursue informed decisions. Nourishment proficiency, the capacity to comprehend and apply sustenance data, is a vital determinant of dietary way of behaving. Thorough sustenance training programs, beginning from youth and going on all through the life expectancy, outfit people with the information and abilities to explore the intricate scene of food decisions.

The job of policymakers in establishing a climate that upholds a reasonable eating routine is significant. Regulation and strategies that elevate admittance to quality food sources, control food showcasing, and give nourishment schooling add to forming a food climate helpful for wellbeing. The execution of drives, for example, food marking, menu straightforwardness, and tax collection on undesirable food sources lines up with worldwide endeavors to address the rising tide of diet-related illnesses.

3.2 Discussing the role of macronutrients and micronutrients

The job of macronutrients and micronutrients in the human eating regimen is essential for keeping up with wellbeing, supporting physiological capabilities, and forestalling wholesome lacks. These fundamental parts, which incorporate sugars, proteins, fats, nutrients, and minerals, are major to the body's development, energy creation, and by and large prosperity.

Macronutrients comprise the heft of the eating routine and give the energy important to day to day exercises. Carbs, the essential wellspring of energy, are found in food varieties like grains, organic products, and vegetables. These mixtures are separated into glucose, which fills in as a fuel for the body's cells, especially the cerebrum and muscles. The consideration of mind boggling starches, like entire grains and vegetables, guarantees a supported arrival of energy and controls glucose levels.

Proteins, made out of amino acids, are basic for building and fixing tissues. Found in sources like meat, poultry, fish, eggs, dairy items, and plant-based food sources like beans and lentils, proteins assume assorted parts in the body. Catalysts, antibodies, chemicals, and primary parts like muscles and skin all depend on proteins for their development and capability. A reasonable eating routine incorporates a sufficient admission of different protein sources to meet the body's prerequisites for fundamental amino acids.

Fats, frequently disparaged however fundamental for wellbeing, are another macronutrient with complex jobs. Sound fats, for example, monounsaturated and polyunsaturated fats tracked down in olive oil, avocados, nuts, and greasy fish, add to cell structure, chemical creation, and the retention of fat-solvent nutrients (A, D, E, and K). Adjusting various kinds of fats and staying away from over the top soaked and trans fats is pivotal for supporting cardiovascular wellbeing.

While macronutrients give the energy expected to everyday working, micronutrients are fundamental for keeping up with wellbeing at the cell and biochemical levels. Nutrients and minerals, by and large known as micronutrients, assume explicit and frequently synergistic parts in different physiological cycles.

Nutrients are natural mixtures expected in modest quantities for explicit capabilities. L-ascorbic acid, for example, is fundamental for collagen combination, wound mending, and resistant capability. Citrus natural products, berries, and vegetables are rich wellsprings of L-ascorbic acid. Vitamin D, significant for bone wellbeing and calcium assimilation, is combined by the skin in light of daylight and can likewise be gotten from strengthened food varieties or enhancements. The B-nutrients, including B1 (thiamine), B2 (riboflavin), B3 (niacin), B6 (pyridoxine), B12 (cobalamin), and folate, are associated with energy digestion, nerve capability, and DNA combination, with food sources going from entire grains and salad greens to meat and dairy.

Minerals are inorganic components that serve different capabilities in the body. Calcium, tracked down in dairy items, mixed greens, and braced food varieties, is fundamental for bone wellbeing, muscle capability, and blood coagulating. Iron, present in meats, vegetables, and braced oats, is essential for oxygen transport in the blood. Zinc, tracked down in meat, dairy, and vegetables, upholds safe capability and wound recuperating. Sodium and potassium, significant for liquid equilibrium and nerve capability, are tracked down in different food varieties, with an accentuation on natural products, vegetables, and entire grains for potassium and control in salt admission for sodium.

The interchange among macronutrients and micronutrients features the intricacy of dietary prerequisites. Accomplishing an equilibrium in the admission of sugars, proteins, and fats, alongside an adequate stockpile of nutrients and minerals, is pivotal for meeting the body's different nourishing requirements.

Prescription For A Healthy Life

The meaning of macronutrients and micronutrients stretches out past simple food to preventive and helpful jobs in wellbeing. A lack or overabundance of these fundamental parts can prompt a scope of medical problems. For example, lacking calcium admission might bring about debilitated bones and an expanded gamble of cracks, while inadequate iron can prompt sickliness, portrayed by exhaustion and shortcoming.

Then again, an abundance of certain macronutrients or micronutrients might add to medical conditions. High admission of soaked fats and cholesterol is related with an expanded gamble of cardiovascular infection, while extreme sodium utilization might add to hypertension. Additionally, consuming an overabundance of specific nutrients or minerals through supplements without clinical direction can prompt poisonousness and unfriendly wellbeing impacts.

The idea of bioavailability adds one more layer of intricacy to supplement retention and usage. Bioavailability alludes to the degree and rate at which a supplement is retained and utilized by the body. Factors like the type of the supplement in food, the presence of different supplements, and individual contrasts in digestion can impact bioavailability. For instance, the iron in plant-based food sources (non-heme iron) is less promptly assimilated than the iron in meat (heme iron). Joining non-heme iron sources with L-ascorbic acid rich food varieties can improve assimilation.

Dietary examples and social practices additionally impact the accessibility and admission of macronutrients and micronutrients. Local weight control plans might include explicit food sources that are rich wellsprings of specific supplements. For example, a customary Mediterranean eating routine is portrayed by an overflow of natural products, vegetables, olive oil, and fish, giving an abundance of nutrients, minerals, and solid fats. Social inclinations, food restrictions, and neighborhood farming practices add to the variety of supplement sources in various populaces.

With regards to general wellbeing, tending to unhealthiness requires a complex methodology. While ailing health is frequently connected with undernutrition, described by inadequate admission of calories and fundamental supplements, overnutrition is a similarly squeezing concern. Overnutrition, driven by unreasonable calorie admission, unfortunate dietary decisions, and stationary ways of life, adds to the worldwide ascent in stoutness and diet-related sicknesses.

Micronutrient lacks, otherwise called secret yearning, represent a one of a kind test. Indeed, even in situations where caloric admission is adequate, an absence of explicit nutrients and minerals can prompt medical problems. Endeavors to battle stowed away craving include food fortress, supplementation, and general wellbeing drives to advance different and supplement rich weight control plans. For example, invigorating staple food varieties like flour with folic corrosive aides address folate inadequacies, especially significant for forestalling brain tube surrenders during pregnancy.

The job of macronutrients and micronutrients in supporting resistant capability is especially applicable, given the worldwide spotlight on wellbeing and prosperity. Sufficient sustenance is critical for keeping a powerful resistant reaction, with different supplements assuming explicit parts in safe capability. L-ascorbic acid, found in citrus products of the soil, has cancer prevention agent properties and supports resistant cell capability. Vitamin D, combined through daylight openness and tracked down in greasy fish and sustained food varieties, is fundamental for safe guideline. Zinc, got from meat, dairy, and vegetables, is associated with insusceptible cell action and immune response creation.

The connection among sustenance and safe capability has acquired unmistakable quality, particularly with regards to irresistible sicknesses. While nourishment alone can't forestall or fix contaminations, an even eating routine adds to in general wellbeing and flexibility. Healthful help is many times a urgent part of clinical mediations, especially in instances of unhealthiness or explicit supplement lacks.

The unique idea of nourishment research persistently reveals new bits of knowledge into the unpredictable cooperations among supplements and the human body. Nutrigenomics, a field at the crossing point of nourishment and hereditary qualities, investigates how individual hereditary varieties impact reactions to dietary parts. This customized way to deal with nourishment perceives that people might have remarkable supplement necessities in view of their hereditary cosmetics. Hereditary variables can impact supplement digestion, assimilation, and usage, forming individual reactions to dietary mediations.

The effect of macronutrients and micronutrients on psychological well-being is a developing area of examination. The stomach cerebrum hub, a bidirectional correspondence network between the stomach and the focal sensory system, highlights the association among diet and mental prosperity.

Arising proof proposes that the stomach microbiota, impacted by diet, may assume a part in psychological wellness problems, including tension and discouragement. Explicit supplements, like omega-3 unsaturated fats and certain nutrients, possibly affect state of mind and mental capability.

In the domain of sports sustenance, the job of macronutrients takes on added importance. Competitors have special energy and supplement prerequisites, affected by variables like preparation force, term, and individual metabolic rates. Sugars are an essential wellspring of energy for perseverance exercises, while protein assumes a significant part in muscle fix and recuperation. Sufficient hydration, alongside electrolytes like sodium and potassium, is fundamental for keeping up with liquid equilibrium during actual effort.

The reconciliation of nourishing standards into medical services is principal for forestalling and overseeing different ailments. Clinical sustenance treatment, a remedial methodology that utilizes dietary mediations to treat and oversee illnesses, has turned into a foundation in medical services practice. Conditions like diabetes, cardiovascular sickness, and hunger can frequently be actually overseen through designated dietary techniques, diminishing the dependence on pharmacological therapies.

3.3 Providing practical tips for healthy eating and meal planning

Smart dieting and feast arranging are key parts of an even way of life that adds to in general wellbeing and prosperity. Taking on nutritious dietary propensities includes going with careful decisions, taking into account an assortment of nutritional categories, and guaranteeing that dinners give fundamental supplements in proper extents. This down to earth guide means to offer noteworthy hints for people hoping to upgrade their dietary patterns and foster compelling dinner arranging procedures.

Embrace a Decent Eating routine:

Focus on a decent eating routine that incorporates various food varieties from various nutrition types. Center around integrating organic products, vegetables, entire grains, lean proteins, and sound fats into your feasts. This variety guarantees that you get an expansive range of fundamental supplements, advancing generally wellbeing and forestalling nourishing lacks.

Segment Control:

Be aware of part sizes to abstain from gorging. Utilize more modest plates, bowls, and utensils to assist with controlling parts. Pay attention to your body's craving and completion prompts, and go for the gold that fulfill your wholesome necessities without unnecessary caloric admission.

Hydration is Critical:

Remain enough hydrated by drinking a lot of water over the course of the day. Water is fundamental for assimilation, supplement retention, and generally prosperity. Limit sweet refreshments and settle on water, home grown teas, or implanted water with leafy foods for added character.

Incorporate Different Tones:

The energetic shades of foods grown from the ground show a rich exhibit of nutrients, minerals, and cell reinforcements. Plan to remember a range of varieties for your feasts to guarantee a different scope of supplements. This not just improves the wholesome profile of your eating regimen yet additionally adds visual enticement for your plate.

Focus on Entire Food sources:

Pick entire, insignificantly handled food varieties over exceptionally handled and refined choices. Entire food sources, like organic products, vegetables, entire grains, nuts, and seeds, hold their regular supplements and fiber content. This supports ideal processing, gives supported energy, and adds to long haul wellbeing.

Careful Eating:

Practice careful eating by appreciating each nibble and focusing on the tangible experience of your dinners. Keep away from interruptions like electronic gadgets while eating, and pay attention to your body's yearning and completion prompts. This cultivates a better relationship with food and advances a more noteworthy appreciation for the eating experience.

Feast Preparing for Progress:
Plan and get ready feasts ahead of time to make smart dieting more helpful. Put away opportunity every week to hack vegetables, cook grains, and pre-segment snacks. Having nutritious choices promptly accessible decreases the compulsion to depend on less solid decisions during active times.

Incorporate Lean Proteins:
Integrate lean protein sources into your dinners to help muscle wellbeing, satiety, and by and large prosperity. Instances of lean proteins incorporate poultry, fish, tofu, vegetables, and low-fat dairy items. Shifting protein sources adds variety to your eating regimen and guarantees a complete amino corrosive profile.

Pick Sound Fats:
Decide on wellsprings of solid fats, like avocados, nuts, seeds, and olive oil. These fats add to heart wellbeing, support supplement retention, and give a sensation of satiety. Limit the admission of immersed and trans fats tracked down in handled and broiled food sources.

Peruse Food Names:
Look into food marks to pursue informed decisions about the items you devour. Focus on serving sizes, supplement content, and the fixing list. Search for food sources with insignificant added substances, lower added sugars, and restricted immersed fats.

Limit Added Sugars:
Decrease the utilization of food sources and refreshments high in added sugars. This incorporates sweet beverages, confections, and handled snacks. Choose regular wellsprings of pleasantness, like organic products, and be aware of stowed away sugars in bundled food sources.

Integrate Entire Grains:
Pick entire grains over refined grains for improved healthy benefit. Entire grains, like earthy colored rice, quinoa, oats, and entire wheat, give fiber, nutrients, and minerals. This balances out glucose levels, upholds processing, and adds to long haul wellbeing.

Enhance Cooking Strategies:
Investigate different cooking strategies to improve the flavor and nourishing nature of your feasts. Try different things with barbecuing, simmering, steaming, sautéing, and baking. Every strategy offers a remarkable culinary encounter and permits you to partake in a scope of surfaces and flavors.

Pay attention to Your Body:
Focus on yearning and completion prompts, and eat when you are ravenous. Stay away from prohibitive weight control plans or eating designs that might

prompt sensations of hardship. A manageable way to deal with good dieting includes partaking in a wide assortment of food varieties with some restraint.

Nibble Astutely:
Pick supplement thick tidbits that give supported energy between feasts. Choices like new natural product, yogurt, nuts, and vegetable sticks with hummus are healthy decisions. Be aware of piece measures and select tidbits that line up with your healthful objectives.

Limit Handled Food varieties:
Limit the admission of exceptionally handled food varieties that are many times high in undesirable fats, sodium, and added substances. These food varieties add to abundance calorie consumption without giving significant healthful advantages. All things considered, center around entire, supplement rich choices.

Be Adaptable and Appreciate Treats With some restraint:
Take on an adaptable way to deal with your eating routine that considers intermittent treats. Partaking in your #1 food sources with some restraint is a feasible method for keeping a sound connection with eating. Hardship frequently prompts desires and may ruin long haul adherence to a nutritious eating regimen.

Think about Dietary Inclinations and Limitations:
Tailor your feast intend to oblige any dietary inclinations or limitations you might have. Whether you follow a veggie lover, vegetarian, sans gluten, or other explicit dietary example, plan dinners that line up with your singular requirements while guaranteeing a decent supplement consumption.

Incorporate Aged Food varieties:
Integrate aged food varieties into your eating regimen to advance stomach well-being. Yogurt, kefir, sauerkraut, kimchi, and miso are instances of aged food sources that contain helpful probiotics. These microorganisms support a good arrangement of stomach microscopic organisms and add to stomach related prosperity.

Remain Informed and Look for Proficient Direction:
Remain informed about sustenance by perusing respectable sources, remaining refreshed on dietary rules, and taking into account the most recent examination. In the event that you have explicit wellbeing concerns or objectives, talk with an enlisted dietitian or medical care proficient who can give customized direction in view of your singular necessities.

Mind the Timing:
Consider the planning of your dinners and snacks to keep up with reliable energy levels over the course of the day. Hold back nothing, feasts and consolidate solid tidbits when expected to forestall exorbitant appetite and gorging later in the day.

Take part in Dinner Variety:
Embrace a different scope of cooking styles and flavors to keep your dinners fascinating and pleasant. Explore different avenues regarding worldwide recipes,

flavors, and spices to change up your eating regimen. This improves the tactile experience of eating as well as widens your healthful admission.

Limit Handled Meats:
Decrease the admission of handled meats, like frankfurters, bacon, and shop meats, which might be high in sodium and unfortunate fats. Pick lean, natural protein sources like poultry, fish, and vegetables as choices.

Plan and Shop Admirably:
Before shopping for food, plan your feasts for the week and make a shopping list in light of your arranged recipes. This assists you with keeping fixed on buying nutritious food varieties and limits the compulsion to purchase undesirable tidbits or drive things.

Investigate Plant-Based Choices:
Coordinate plant-based feasts into your eating routine to expand protein sources and increment your admission of plant food varieties. This can incorporate dinners revolved around vegetables, tofu, tempeh, or integrating more vegetables into customary dishes.

Construct a Strong Climate:
Encircle yourself with a strong climate that energizes good dieting. Share your dietary objectives with family or companions, and think about preparing or sharing dinners together. A strong local area can encourage positive propensities and make good dieting more charming.

Remain Predictable with Actual work:
Standard actual work supplements good dieting by supporting in general prosperity. Participate in exercises you appreciate, whether it's strolling, cycling, moving, or taking part in sports. Active work adds to a sound way of life as well as lifts temperament and energy levels.

Practice Natural Eating:
Tune into your body's normal yearning and completion signals and practice natural eating. Permit yourself to partake in various food sources without responsibility, and perceive the significance of both feeding your body and appreciating the joys of eating.

Limit Fluid Calories:
Be aware of fluid calories from sweet refreshments, cocktails, and fatty espresso drinks. Select water, home grown teas, or dark espresso as essential refreshment decisions and save sweet or fatty beverages for incidental treats.

Alter Recipes for Wellbeing:
Alter recipes to make them more nutritious without forfeiting flavor. Trade out elements for better other options, for example, utilizing entire grain flour, lessening added sugars, or integrating more vegetables into dishes.

Observe Food as a Social Encounter:

Prescription For A Healthy Life

Food isn't just sustenance yet additionally a social encounter. Celebrate feasts with loved ones, and partake in the social and social parts of sharing food. This upgrades the delight of eating and encourages positive relationship with nutritious decisions.

Keep Solid Snacks Available:
Stock your storage space and cooler with sound nibble choices to decrease the allurement of going after less nutritious decisions. Having advantageous and nutritious snacks promptly accessible settles on it more straightforward to pursue sound choices between dinners.

Plan for Unique Events:
On unique events or during get-togethers, prepare for extravagances without feeling remorseful. Partake in the festival and return to your normal dietary patterns subsequently. A fair and adaptable methodology considers incidental treats while keeping a solid generally speaking eating routine.

Focus on Fiber-Rich Food varieties:
Incorporate fiber-rich food sources, like organic products, vegetables, entire grains, vegetables, and nuts, to help stomach related wellbeing. Fiber adds to satiety, manages glucose levels, and advances a sound stomach microbiota.

Investigate Careful Cooking:
Take part in careful cooking by focusing on the fixings, readiness process, and the tangible parts of cooking. This care stretches out to the delight in the completed feast, cultivating a more profound association with the food you eat.

Limit Exceptionally Handled Tidbits:
Limit the admission of profoundly handled tidbits that are many times high in salt, sugar, and undesirable fats. All things being equal, pick supplement thick bites that add to your general supplement admission and backing your wellbeing objectives.

Try different things with Spices and Flavors:
Improve the kind of your dinners without depending on inordinate salt or added sugars by exploring different avenues regarding spices and flavors. New spices, garlic, ginger, and various flavors can raise the flavor of your dishes while giving extra medical advantages.

Make a Daily schedule:
Lay out a supper time schedule that works for your timetable. Consistency in dinner timing directs hunger and forestalls whimsical eating designs. Plan normal dinners and snacks to guarantee a consistent stock of energy over the course of the day.

Think about Food Responsive qualities:
Know about any food responsive qualities or sensitivities you might have, and change your dinner plan in like manner. On the off chance that you suspect explicit

responsive qualities, talk with a medical services proficient or enlisted dietitian for direction on recognizing and overseeing them.

Observe Progress, Not Flawlessness:

Center around progress as opposed flawlessly in your excursion toward better eating. Celebrate little triumphs, recognize positive changes, and perceive that building practical propensities requires some investment. Embrace the growing experience and be caring to yourself en route.

Integrating these functional tips into your regular routine can add to a more careful and wellbeing elevating way to deal with eating. Good dieting is a dynamic and individualized excursion, and finding an offset that lines up with your inclinations, way of life, and nourishing necessities is critical. By embracing these techniques, you can develop a positive relationship with food, support your general prosperity, and establish the groundwork for long haul wellbeing and imperativeness.

Chapter 4

The Power of Exercise

The force of activity is a diverse power that rises above the limits of actual wellbeing, expanding its impact into the domains of mental prosperity, close to home equilibrium, and, surprisingly, mental capability. From the musical thump of a sprinter's heart to the controlled accuracy of a weightlifter's developments, practice is a unique ensemble that coordinates a horde of physiological reactions inside the human body.

At its center, practice is a physiological boost that sets off an outpouring of versatile reactions. The cardiovascular framework, contained the heart and veins, goes through exceptional changes during exercise. As the interest for oxygen-rich blood floods, the heart siphons all the more vivaciously, proficiently conveying this crucial asset to working muscles. The corridors expand to oblige expanded blood stream, guaranteeing that oxygen and supplements arrive at each side of the body. This upgraded cardiovascular proficiency upholds quick execution as well as adds to long haul cardiovascular wellbeing.

At the same time, the respiratory framework enhances its endeavors. The lungs, similar to howls, extend and agreement to augment the trading of oxygen and carbon dioxide. With every breath, the body breathes in life-supporting oxygen and ousts metabolic results. This many-sided dance between the cardiovascular and respiratory frameworks is the physiological pith of vigorous activity, a foundation of actual wellness.

However, the impact of activity stretches out past the actual domain. Taking part in standard actual work has been connected to a heap of emotional wellbeing benefits. The arrival of endorphins, frequently alluded to as the "vibe great" chemicals, is a notable result of activity. These neurochemicals go about as normal mind-set enhancers, easing pressure and advancing a feeling of prosperity. In the pains of a difficult exercise, people might encounter an euphoric state regularly known as the "sprinter's high." This psychological elevate isn't just a brief sensation however a demonstration of the significant effect of activity on emotional wellness.

Additionally, practice has been displayed to moderate the side effects of tension and misery. The cadenced, monotonous nature of numerous proactive tasks prompts a reflective state, quieting the brain and lessening the hold of concerns. The physiological changes going with work out, for example, expanded blood stream to the cerebrum and the arrival of synapses like serotonin, add to a climate helpful for psychological wellness.

Notwithstanding its job in mental prosperity, practice arises as an integral asset for stress the executives. The requests of present day life frequently subject people to persistent pressure, a condition with impeding consequences for both mental and actual wellbeing. Standard activity goes about as a counterforce, giving an outlet to repressed pressure and advancing a condition of unwinding. Whether through the cadenced beating of running shoes on a path or the purposeful progression of yoga presents, people track down comfort in actual work, a relief from the bedlam of day to day existence.

Past psychological well-being, practice is a foundation of keeping a sound body weight and forestalling corpulence — a worldwide wellbeing concern. The cutting edge way of life, portrayed by stationary ways of behaving and an overflow of calorie-thick food varieties, has added to an ascent in heftiness rates. Work out, related to a reasonable eating routine, turns into a strong device for weight the board. It consumes calories during the movement as well as improves metabolic rate, prompting expanded calorie consumption even very still. The blend of high-impact practice for cardiovascular wellbeing and obstruction preparing to fabricate slender bulk makes an all encompassing way to deal with weight the executives.

Besides, practice assumes a vital part in forming body organization. Obstruction preparing, incorporating exercises like weightlifting and bodyweight works out, invigorates the development and support of slender bulk. This adds to a conditioned physical make-up as well as expands the body's metabolic limit.

Muscle tissue is metabolically dynamic, requiring more energy for upkeep than fat tissue. Hence, people with a higher extent of fit bulk will generally have a higher basal metabolic rate, working with weight the executives.

The advantages of activity reach out to metabolic wellbeing, especially with regards to insulin responsiveness. Insulin, a chemical delivered by the pancreas, assumes a significant part in managing glucose levels. In states of insulin opposition, cells become less receptive to the activities of insulin, prompting raised glucose levels — a sign of type 2 diabetes. Normal activity upgrades insulin awareness, permitting cells to proficiently take-up glucose from the circulation system. This brings down the gamble of creating diabetes as well as helps in the administration of existing circumstances.

Besides, practice applies a significant impact on bone wellbeing. Weight-bearing and obstruction practices invigorate bone rebuilding, upgrading bone thickness and strength. This is especially vital in the counteraction of osteoporosis, a condition portrayed by weak and delicate bones. As people age, the gamble of osteoporosis increments, making weight-bearing activities an essential part of keeping up with skeletal wellbeing.

The advantages of activity are not selective to grown-ups; they stretch out to the formative long periods of young life and immaturity. Actual work during these early stages is related with worked on scholastic execution, improved mental capability, and the foundation of long lasting wellbeing propensities. Past the actual advantages, commitment to sports and proactive tasks cultivates interactive abilities, collaboration, and a feeling of discipline among the young.

With regards to maturing, practice arises as a strong partner in the battle against age-related decline. The maturing system is joined by a progressive loss of bulk and strength, a peculiarity known as sarcopenia. Customary opposition preparing, combined with sufficient protein consumption, balances this decay, protecting bulk and practical limit. Also, practice has been connected to mental wellbeing in more seasoned grown-ups, with actual work displayed to decrease the gamble of mental degradation and neurodegenerative sicknesses.

As the comprehension of activity science advances, so does the acknowledgment of its effect on invulnerable capability. Standard, moderate-force practice has been related with a decreased gamble of contaminations, including respiratory diseases. The resistant supporting impacts of activity are believed to be intervened by different components, like the advancement of mitigating reactions and the assembly of safe cells all through the body. In any case, it's pivotal to figure out some kind of harmony, as extreme activity, particularly at focused energies, may briefly stifle safe capability.

Chasing in general wellbeing and prosperity, it's fundamental to perceive that the advantages of activity are not bound to a particular sort or power. The critical lies in finding exercises that line up with individual inclinations, interests, and actual abilities.

Whether it's the cadenced progression of a dance class, the isolation of a long run, or the brotherhood of group activities, the range of activity is different, taking special care of the exceptional requirements and inclinations of people.

Also, the idea of activity reaches out past the organized schedules of the rec center or the track. Integrating actual work into day to day existence through exercises like strolling, cycling, or cultivating adds to aggregate medical advantages. The cutting edge inactive way of life, described by delayed times of sitting, has been recognized as a huge wellbeing risk. Consequently, the advancement of a functioning way of life, which incorporates both arranged practice meetings and coincidental active work, is essential for by and large wellbeing.

The impact of activity on smartness and mental capability is an area of developing interest and exploration. The cerebrum, frequently viewed as the war room of the body, isn't excluded from the impacts of active work. Studies have exhibited that activity, especially oxygen consuming activity, upgrades mental capability, including memory, consideration, and chief capability. The expanded blood stream to the mind, the arrival of neurotrophic factors, and the advancement of brain adaptability are among the instruments that underlie the mental advantages of activity.

Besides, practice has been investigated as an expected mediation for state of mind issues and mental degradation. In conditions like Alzheimer's sickness, where mental degradation is a trademark, standard active work has shown guarantee in easing back the movement of side effects. The multifaceted transaction between the body and the cerebrum, intervened by the neurobiological impacts of activity, highlights the all encompassing nature of wellbeing.

In the domain of preventive medication, practice remains as an impressive safeguard against a range of ongoing sicknesses. Cardiovascular sicknesses, incorporating conditions like coronary illness and stroke, are among the main sources of worldwide bleakness and mortality. Standard activity, with its cardiovascular advantages, is a powerful preventive measure against these circumstances. It adds to the support of sound pulse, cholesterol levels, and by and large cardiovascular capability.

The relationship among exercise and disease anticipation is one more area of dynamic examination. While the relationship is intricate and changes across various disease types, proof proposes that ordinary active work is related with a diminished gamble of specific malignant growths. The systems fundamental this defensive impact incorporate the tweak of hormonal levels, the guideline of irritation, and the improvement of safe reconnaissance.

Besides, practice assumes a critical part in the administration and recovery of persistent illnesses. Conditions like diabetes, joint pain, and persistent obstructive aspiratory infection (COPD) benefit from the consideration of custom fitted activity programs. Practice turns into a restorative device, further developing side effects, upgrading useful limit, and adding to a general improvement in personal satisfaction for people with constant circumstances.

In the steadily advancing scene of wellbeing and wellness, the job of practice in molding body piece has collected critical consideration. Past the numbers on a scale, body organization mirrors the extent of fit bulk to fat tissue. While weight the board includes caloric equilibrium, body creation is impacted by the sort of calories consumed and the idea of actual work.

Opposition preparing, described by exercises that challenge the muscles against outer obstruction, is a foundation of body organization the board. Not at all like high-impact work out, which fundamentally consumes calories during the movement, obstruction preparing prompts a delayed height in metabolic rate post-work out. This peculiarity, known as abundance post-practice oxygen utilization (EPOC), adds to calorie consumption past the exercise meeting.

The quest for tasteful objectives, like muscle definition and conditioning, frequently includes a mix of obstruction preparing and cardiovascular activity. The cooperative energy between these modalities tends to both the protection of fit bulk and the decrease of muscle to fat ratio. While feel are emotional and differ among people, the comprehensive way to deal with wellbeing, including both capability and structure, stays a core value.

The coordination of innovation into the domain of activity has introduced another time of customized wellness. Wellness trackers, smartwatches, and portable applications furnish people with constant input on their active work, considering a more nuanced comprehension of their wellness process. These mechanical apparatuses not just screen key measurements, for example, pulse, steps taken, and calories consumed yet in addition offer experiences into rest designs, feelings of anxiety, and in general prosperity.

Virtual stages and online work out regimes have democratized admittance to master direction and various exercise routine schedules. From virtual yoga classes to intelligent wellness applications, people can browse a plenty of choices that line up with their inclinations and objectives. The gamification of wellness, where clients participate in difficulties, procure rewards, and keep tabs on their development, adds a component of tomfoolery and inspiration to the activity experience.

While innovation works with comfort and openness, it is crucial for find some kind of harmony and keep an association with the basic parts of active work. The straightforwardness of binding up running shoes for a run or taking part in bodyweight practices requires negligible hardware and highlights the immortal idea of activity. The pith of active work lies in the delight of development, the association among psyche and body, and the quest for wellbeing past mathematical measurements.

In the mission for ideal wellbeing, sustenance and exercise join as indistinguishable partners. The connection between dietary decisions and active work is bidirectional, each impacting the other in a unique dance of equilibrium.

Satisfactory sustenance powers the body for ideal execution during exercise, while the metabolic requests of actual work shape nourishing necessities.

The idea of "energizing for the exercise" includes key dietary decisions to help energy levels, upgrade execution, and work with recuperation. Carbs, the body's favored energy source, assume a focal part in this perspective. Consuming sugars before practice gives promptly accessible fuel, while post-practice sustenance recharges glycogen stores and works with muscle recuperation. Protein, fundamental for muscle fix and development, expects importance in the post-practice period.

Hydration, frequently disregarded at this point basic, is a foundation of activity execution. Lack of hydration can disable physical and mental capability, compromise perseverance, and impede recuperation. Liquid requirements change among people and are impacted by variables like environment, practice force, and individual perspiration rates. Checking hydration status and taking on customized techniques to keep up with liquid equilibrium are fundamental parts of a thorough way to deal with work out.

In the more extensive setting of wellbeing and life span, the entwining of sustenance and exercise reaches out to the idea of caloric equilibrium. Accomplishing a harmony between caloric admission and use is principal for weight the board. While practice adds to caloric use, dietary decisions impact the energy condition. The nature of calories devoured, including the equilibrium of macronutrients and the incorporation of micronutrient-rich food sources, shapes weight as well as generally speaking wellbeing.

The harmonious connection among sustenance and exercise turns out to be especially significant with regards to execution competitors. Perseverance competitors, strength competitors, and those participated in focused energy preparing have particular nourishing requirements custom-made to their particular requests. Periodization of nourishment, adjusting dietary techniques to preparing cycles, turns into an essential device for improving execution, supporting recuperation, and forestalling overtraining.

Chasing after wellbeing and wellness, the mental parts of activity structure a vital part. Inspiration, frequently viewed as the main impetus behind conduct, expects a focal job in supporting a reliable work-out daily practice. Persuasive elements shift among people and may incorporate inborn variables, like an individual pride, and outward factors, including outer prizes or social acknowledgment.

The mental advantages of activity stretch out past inspiration, including pressure the executives, further developed state of mind, and upgraded mental capability. The demonstration of putting forth and accomplishing wellness objectives gives a feeling of inspiration and achievement.

The development of a positive outlook, strength even with difficulties, and an appreciation for the excursion add to the psychological determination that goes with a normal work-out daily practice.

Nonetheless, the mental scene of activity isn't resistant to challenges. Hindrances to work out, going from time limitations to saw absence of capacity, may hinder commencement and adherence to actual work. Beating these boundaries requires a customized approach, recognizing individual inclinations, tending to mental hindrances, and encouraging a strong climate.

The social component of activity further highlights its effect on in general prosperity. Bunch wellness classes, group activities, and exercise networks make a feeling of having a place and kinship. The common quest for wellness objectives, the consolation of friends, and the aggregate energy of a gathering add to a positive and spurring exercise insight.

Conversely, the isolation of singular exercises, like running or weightlifting, offers a space for contemplation and self-disclosure. The musical rhythm of strides or the clunking of loads turns into a reflective soundtrack, permitting people to interface with their viewpoints and feelings. The variety of activity modalities, each offering an interesting mix of social cooperation and contemplation, takes care of the differed inclinations of people.

With regards to general wellbeing, the advancement of active work arises as a cultural goal. The worldwide weight of non-transferable infections, including cardiovascular illnesses, diabetes, and stoutness, highlights the requirement for extensive preventive systems. Actual latency, recognized as a modifiable gamble factor, contributes fundamentally to the ascent in these medical issue.

4.1 Exploring the benefits of regular physical activity

Customary active work is a foundation of a sound way of life, offering a large number of advantages that stretch out past actual prosperity. From working on cardiovascular wellbeing to upgrading mental flexibility, the positive effect of customary activity is broad and multi-layered. In this investigation, we dig into the different elements of how taking part in steady active work adds to by and large wellbeing, both genuinely and intellectually.

At its center, customary actual work is instrumental in keeping a sound cardiovascular framework. The heart, being a muscle, turns out to be more proficient and strong with ordinary activity. As people take part in exercises that hoist their pulse, the heart adjusts by siphoning blood all the more proficiently, which, thusly, further develops dissemination. This expanded proficiency lessens the gamble of cardiovascular illnesses, for example, respiratory failures and strokes. Moreover, actual work directs pulse, keeping it inside a sound reach and limiting the burden on the heart.

Past the cardiovascular advantages, normal activity assumes an essential part in weight the board. In this present reality where stationary ways of life and undesirable dietary propensities add to an ascent in corpulence, active work turns into a urgent device in fighting overabundance weight. Taking part in practices that consume calories supports weight reduction as well as assists in keeping a sound body with weighting. This, thusly, decreases the gamble of corpulence related conditions, including type 2 diabetes, certain diseases, and joint issues.

The positive effect of active work stretches out to outer muscle wellbeing, cultivating solid bones and versatile muscles. Weight-bearing activities, like strolling, running, and opposition preparing, animate the unresolved issues denser, which is especially significant in forestalling osteoporosis, a condition described by delicate bones. Simultaneously, muscles that are consistently participated in active work become more grounded and more adaptable, lessening the gamble of wounds and working on in general versatility.

Notwithstanding the actual advantages, standard actual work altogether adds to psychological wellness and prosperity. Practice has been shown to be a strong counteractant to stress, uneasiness, and melancholy. At the point when people participate in active work, the body discharges endorphins, frequently alluded to as "happy go lucky" chemicals, which go about as normal state of mind lifters. This compound response eases pressure as well as advances a feeling of prosperity and unwinding.

Also, the mental advantages of customary activity are progressively perceived. Active work has been connected to worked on mental capability, including better memory, more honed center, and improved inventiveness. This is credited to the expanded blood stream to the cerebrum during exercise, which sustains the neurons and advances the development of new associations. In the long haul, customary actual work might try and assume a part in diminishing the gamble of neurodegenerative circumstances like Alzheimer's sickness.

In the cutting edge age, where stationary positions and screen-driven ways of life have turned into the standard, the significance of integrating actual work into everyday schedules couldn't possibly be more significant. Inactive conduct has been related with a plenty of wellbeing chances, including weight, cardiovascular infections, and metabolic issues. In this manner, separating delayed times of sitting with short explosions of actual work, like extending or strolling, is vital for generally wellbeing.

One angle frequently neglected in conversations about actual work is its part in advancing quality rest. The connection among exercise and rest is bidirectional - normal actual work further develops rest quality, and thusly, sufficient rest upgrades the body's capacity to take part in proactive tasks. Practice controls rest designs by advancing the arrival of melatonin, the chemical liable for rest enlistment. Besides, it decreases side effects of a sleeping disorder and rest apnea, adding to a relaxing and helpful night's rest.

With regards to persistent sicknesses, active work arises as a preventive and helpful measure. Conditions like sort 2 diabetes, hypertension, and certain tumors are firmly connected to way of life factors, including diet and active work. Participating in ordinary activity controls glucose levels, oversee pulse, and decrease the gamble of fostering particular sorts of malignant growths. For people previously living with persistent circumstances, active work is much of the time a vital part of their administration and recovery plans.

As social orders wrestle with the rising pervasiveness of psychological wellness issues, perceiving the job of actual work in mental prosperity becomes principal. Practice is viewed as a proof based mediation for different emotional well-being conditions, including gloom and uneasiness problems. The helpful impacts of active work are not restricted to its effect on synapses; participating in practice likewise gives a feeling of achievement and self-viability, which can be especially enabling for people confronting psychological well-being difficulties.

Social prosperity is one more aspect affected by ordinary actual work. Bunch works out, group activities, and local area based exercises set out open doors for social cooperation and association. These social bonds add to a feeling of having a place and backing, cultivating mental strength and close to home prosperity. The fellowship worked through shared proactive tasks improves interactive abilities and may alleviate sensations of forlornness and disengagement.

A comprehensive comprehension of wellbeing includes the shortfall of disease as well as the presence of positive prosperity. Actual work, with its complex advantages, lines up with this all encompassing viewpoint by tending to different components of wellbeing - physical, mental, and social. The World Wellbeing Association (WHO) perceives the significance of actual work in advancing well-being and suggests no less than 150 minutes of moderate-power or 75 minutes of enthusiastic power practice each week for grown-ups.

The effect of actual work is especially articulated in the domain of preventive medical care. Ordinary activity is a vital calculate forestalling way of life related infections, which represent a huge piece of worldwide grimness and mortality. By embracing a truly dynamic way of life, people can find proactive ways to protect their wellbeing and lessen the weight on medical care frameworks.

Youngsters and teenagers, specifically, stand to benefit fundamentally from customary active work. Actual work is vital to the solid improvement of muscles, bones, and joints. Additionally, it upholds mental turn of events and scholarly execution. Empowering dynamic play and sports cooperation in youthful people not just establishes the groundwork for a solid way of life yet in addition imparts values like collaboration, discipline, and constancy.

In the work environment, the advancement of active work has been connected to further developed efficiency and representative fulfillment. Inactive positions, portrayed by extended periods of time of sitting, have been related with different wellbeing chances, including outer muscle issues and cardiovascular sicknesses. Managers are progressively perceiving the significance of establishing conditions that empower development, for example, giving standing work areas, putting together wellness classes, and advancing dynamic breaks.

The advantages of actual work are not restricted to the individual; they reach out to the local area and society in general. Solid people add to a useful labor force, decreasing non-attendance because of disease. Besides, the financial weight of treating way of life related infections is altogether brought down when deterrent estimates, for example, normal activity are embraced. As people group become more wellbeing cognizant, the stress on medical services frameworks is reduced, and assets can be diverted towards proactive wellbeing advancement.

With regards to maturing, customary active work arises as a strong device for advancing solid maturing and keeping up with freedom. As people age, they might encounter a decrease in bulk, bone thickness, and joint adaptability. Taking part in practices that focus on these angles mitigates age-related declines, saving versatility and utilitarian autonomy. Furthermore, active work has been related with a decreased gamble of mental deterioration in more seasoned grown-ups.

The advantages of actual work stretch out to populaces with constant circumstances, incorporating those with incapacities. Adjusted actual work programs take special care of the extraordinary necessities and capacities of people with inabilities, advancing actual wellness, social cooperation, and in general prosperity. Such projects add to the strengthening and consideration of people who might confront extra hindrances to taking part in standard active work.

While the advantages of actual work are plentiful, it is fundamental to recognize the hindrances that people might look in taking on and keeping a functioning way of life. Financial variables, admittance to safe sporting spaces, and social standards can all impact a singular's capacity to participate in customary active work. Perceiving and tending to these boundaries is pivotal in advancing fair open doors for all people to receive the rewards of active work.

All in all, the investigation of the advantages of customary active work uncovers an embroidery of positive results that range physical, mental, and social elements of wellbeing. From cardiovascular prosperity to mental strength, the effect of activity is significant and sweeping. As people, networks, and social orders embrace the significance of remaining dynamic, the potential for a better and more energetic world turns out to be progressively feasible. The source of inspiration is clear - coordinate active work into everyday schedules.

4.2 Discussing different types of exercises for various fitness levels

Practice is a vital part of a sound way of life, and its viability is in many cases dependent upon fitting exercises to individual wellness levels. Understanding that not all activities are reasonable for everybody, it becomes significant to investigate the range of exercise choices that take special care of assorted wellness levels. Whether you are a novice, halfway, or high level exerciser, the critical lies in picking exercises that line up with your ongoing capacities while offering space for movement.

For fledglings, particularly those new to practice or returning after a delayed break, low-influence exercises are a great beginning stage. These activities are delicate on the joints and limit the gamble of injury, making them available for people with fluctuating degrees of wellness. Strolling is maybe the least difficult and most open type of low-influence work out. It requires no exceptional gear, should be possible practically anyplace, and gives a delicate prologue to cardiovascular movement.

Prescription For A Healthy Life

As well as strolling, swimming is another low-influence practice that offers a full-body exercise. The lightness of water decreases the effect on joints, making it an optimal choice for people with joint pain or joint agony. Swimming connects with numerous muscle gatherings, upgrades cardiovascular wellness, and further develops adaptability. Oceanic vigorous exercise classes further give an organized and pleasant method for integrating low-influence practice into a daily schedule, frequently joined by music and directed developments.

For those slipping into strength preparing, bodyweight practices are a viable and available beginning stage. These activities use the person's own body weight as opposition, requiring negligible gear. Squats, lurches, push-ups, and boards are central bodyweight practices that target significant muscle gatherings. As strength and certainty increment, varieties and movements can be acquainted with ceaselessly challenge the body.

Yoga and Pilates are two trains that consistently mix low-influence developments with care and adaptability. Yoga, with its accentuation on breath control and stances, improves adaptability and advances unwinding. Pilates, then again, centers around center strength and solidness. The two practices offer alterations for various wellness levels, permitting people to advance at their own speed.

As people progress from fledgling to transitional wellness levels, a slow expansion in power and intricacy becomes suitable. Cardiovascular activities, for example, running or running can be presented, gave that legitimate footwear and running surfaces are considered to limit influence on joints. Cycling, whether outside or on an exercise bike, is one more viable method for lifting pulse and fabricate perseverance.

Strength preparing can advance to incorporate free loads or obstruction groups, adding an outer protection from bodyweight works out. Compound activities, like squats, deadlifts, and seat presses, draw in different muscle bunches all the while, enhancing time and productivity. High-intensity exercise, which joins strength and cardio practices in a grouping, offers an extensive exercise that challenges both the cardiovascular and strong frameworks.

Stop and go aerobic exercise (HIIT) is a well known decision for middle of the road exercisers hoping to raise their wellness level. HIIT includes switching back and forth between short explosions of extraordinary movement and times of rest or lower-power work out. This approach works on cardiovascular wellness as well as upgrades metabolic rate, advancing fat misfortune and muscle perseverance. HIIT can be adjusted to different types of activity, including running, cycling, and bodyweight works out.

For those at a middle or high level wellness level, consolidating progressed strength preparing methods turns into a characteristic movement. This might include lifting heavier loads, performing more complicated developments, or consolidating progressed preparing techniques, for example, supersets, drop sets, and pyramids. Working with a guaranteed fitness coach can be valuable at this stage to guarantee legitimate structure, strategy, and program plan.

High level cardiovascular activities might incorporate exercises that request more significant levels of expertise and coordination. Models incorporate kickboxing, paddling, or partaking in focused energy sports like ball or soccer. These exercises challenge the cardiovascular framework as well as give a dynamic and drawing in exercise insight.

Adaptability and portability practices stay significant for people at all wellness levels, yet especially for those at a high level stage. Integrating dynamic stretches, yoga, or designated versatility drills keeps up with joint wellbeing, forestall wounds, and improve generally athletic execution. Customary extending schedules become principal, with an accentuation on accomplishing and keeping a full scope of movement.

Broadly educating, or taking part in different exercises, turns out to be progressively important at cutting edge wellness levels. This approach forestalls abuse wounds, advances generally physicality, and keeps exercises intriguing and testing. A balanced wellness schedule that incorporates a blend of cardiovascular, strength, adaptability, and portability practices guarantees a reasonable and maintainable way to deal with wellness.

While the spotlight up to this point has been on individual activities, the significance of organizing exercises into far reaching schedules ought not be disregarded. The two fledglings and high level people benefit from very much planned exercise programs that address various parts of wellness. This incorporates consolidating a get ready to set up the body for work out, a blend of cardiovascular and strength preparing exercises, and a cool-down to help with recuperation and adaptability.

Notwithstanding wellness level, the rule of movement is vital. Movement includes continuously expanding the force, length, or intricacy of activities to persistently challenge the body and animate variation. This can be accomplished through gradual changes, like adding more weight, expanding exercise recurrence, or consolidating new activities and varieties.

Flexibility is one more basic part of activity at any wellness level. Life conditions, wounds, or changes in wellbeing might require alterations to gym routine schedules. Being available to adjusting the activity routine guarantees that people can keep a reliable and charming way to deal with actual work all through their lives.

It's fundamental to perceive that wellness levels are dynamic and can vary over the long run. Factors, for example, age, way of life changes, and ailments can impact individual wellness levels. Thusly, it's urgent to move toward practice with an outlook that is sensitive to one's ongoing capacities and objectives while staying adaptable and versatile to evolving conditions.

Prescription For A Healthy Life

All in all, the range of activities accessible takes special care of people at different wellness levels, from amateurs setting out on their wellness process to cutting edge exercisers looking for new difficulties. The key is to pick exercises that line up with one's ongoing wellness level, steadily progress in power and intricacy, and embrace a comprehensive methodology that envelops cardiovascular wellness, strength preparing, adaptability, and versatility. By fitting work-out schedules to individual requirements, inclinations, and objectives, people can develop a manageable and long lasting obligation to active work, receiving the various rewards that accompany a functioning and sound way of life.

4.3 Providing a simple exercise routine for readers to follow

Leaving on an excursion to further develop wellness doesn't need to be overpowering or muddled. Laying out a basic yet viable work-out routine can be an incredible beginning stage for people hoping to integrate actual work into their regular routines. The accompanying routine is intended to be open for fledglings while giving a strong groundwork to in general wellness. It incorporates a blend of cardiovascular, strength, and adaptability works out, guaranteeing a balanced way to deal with wellbeing and prosperity.

1. **Warm-up (5-10 minutes):**
   Prior to jumping into additional serious activities, it's essential to heat up the body to plan muscles and joints for development. A powerful warm-up assists increment with blooding stream, adaptability, and by and large internal heat level. Basic warm-up activities might include:
   Walk Set up: Lift your knees towards your chest, swinging your arms in mood.
   Arm Circles: Pivot your arms in little circles, steadily expanding the size.
   Bouncing Jacks: Hop while spreading your legs and arms, then return to the beginning position.
   Bodyweight Squats: Perform squats by bowing your knees and bringing down your hips, then return to a standing position.
2. **Cardiovascular Activity (20-30 minutes):**
   Cardiovascular activity, or cardio, is critical for further developing heart wellbeing, consuming calories, and supporting generally perseverance. Fledglings can begin with moderate-power exercises that lift the pulse without causing inordinate strain. Choices include:
   Energetic Strolling: Stroll at a speed that raises your pulse however permits you to keep a discussion.
   Cycling: Whether outside or on an exercise bike, cycling is a low-influence method for getting the heart siphoning.
   Swimming: A fantastic full-body exercise, swimming is delicate on the joints and gives cardiovascular advantages.

Work out with Rope: A straightforward yet powerful method for lifting the pulse and further develop coordination.

Pick one or a mix of these exercises, going for the gold of 20-30 minutes. As wellness improves, continuously increment the length or force.

3. **Strength Preparing (20-30 minutes, 2-3 times each week):**
   Strength preparing is fundamental for building muscle, further developing digestion, and improving in general useful wellness. Amateurs can begin with bodyweight practices prior to advancing to integrate opposition. An example strength preparing routine might include:

   Bodyweight Squats: 3 arrangements of 10-15 redundancies to focus on the lower body.

   Push-Ups: 3 arrangements of 8-12 redundancies to connect with the chest, shoulders, and rear arm muscles.

   Free weight Lines: Assuming that free weights are accessible, 3 arrangements of 10-12 reiterations for each arm to focus on the back.

   Board: Stand firm on a board footing for 30 seconds to 1 moment to reinforce the center.

   Bodyweight Rushes: 2 arrangements of 10-12 redundancies for each leg to chip away at leg strength and solidness.

   Start with a weight that takes into consideration legitimate structure, steadily expanding obstruction as strength gets to the next level. Strength preparing can be performed 2-3 times each week, considering rest in the middle between.

4. **Adaptability and Extending (10 minutes, day to day):**
   Further developing adaptability upgrades scope of movement, lessens the gamble of wounds, and advances in general joint wellbeing. Integrate extending practices into your daily schedule, zeroing in on significant muscle gatherings. Models include:

   Hamstring Stretch: Sit on the floor with one leg expanded, going after your toes. Hold for 15-30 seconds on every leg.

   Chest Opener: Fasten your hands behind your back, fix your arms, and lift your chest.

   Rear arm muscles Stretch: Bring one arm above, twisting the elbow and arriving at down your back with the contrary hand.

   Quadriceps Stretch: Stand on one leg, bringing the heel towards your hindquarters, and hold for 15-30 seconds on every leg.

   Calf Stretch: Spot one foot forward with a bowed knee and the other foot expanded straight behind you, feeling the stretch in the calf.

   Play out these stretches day to day, particularly after your exercise when your muscles are warm. Hold each stretch for 15-30 seconds, going for the gold and controlled stretch without skipping.

5. **Cool Down (5-10 minutes):**
   Chilling off is crucial for assist the body with changing from practice back to a resting state, forestalling muscle firmness and supporting recuperation. A straightforward cool-down routine might include:
   Strolling or Slow Running: Steadily decline your power to permit your pulse to get back to business as usual.
   Profound Relaxing: Breathe in profoundly through your nose, hold briefly, and breathe out leisurely through your mouth to advance unwinding.
   Delicate Extending: Perform static stretches for significant muscle gatherings, holding each stretch for 15-30 seconds.
6. **Rest and Recuperation:**

Permitting the body time to rest and recuperate is urgent for progress and injury counteraction. Plan no less than a couple of days off rest each week to give your muscles time to fix and revamp. Satisfactory rest, legitimate hydration, and a reasonable eating routine likewise assume crucial parts in supporting generally speaking prosperity and recuperation.

Tips for Progress:

Consistency is Vital: Adhere to your everyday practice, progressively expanding force as your wellness gets to the next level.

Stand by listening to Your Body: Focus on how your body answers work out. Assuming that something feels excruciating (totally unrelated to the inconvenience of testing your muscles), change or avoid the activity.

Remain Hydrated: Hydrate previously, during, and after your exercise to remain hydrated.

Put forth Sensible Objectives: Lay out feasible present moment and long haul objectives to remain roused and keep tabs on your development.

Stir it Up: Keep your routine fascinating by attempting new exercises or shifting the power of your exercises.

Counsel an Expert: In the event that you have any wellbeing concerns or prior conditions, consider talking with a medical services proficient or wellness master prior to beginning another work-out daily schedule.

Keep in mind, the way in to an effective work-out routine is tracking down exercises that you appreciate and that line up with your objectives. Whether it's energetic strolls, strength preparing, or yoga, the main perspective is to make actual work a steady piece of your way of life. As you progress, you can alter and extend your daily practice to keep testing your body and receiving the many rewards of standard activity.

Chapter 5

Mental Health Matters

Psychological wellness is a basic part of generally prosperity, impacting each part of a singular's life. It incorporates close to home, mental, and social prosperity, influencing individuals' thought process, feel, and act. In spite of its significant effect, emotional wellness is in many cases ignored or defamed, thwarting open conversations and deterrent measures. Perceiving the meaning of psychological well-being is the most vital move toward encouraging a general public that qualities and focuses on the prosperity of its individuals.

As of late, there has been a developing familiarity with emotional well-being issues, provoking expanded endeavors to address and destigmatize them. Nonetheless, there is still a lot of work to be finished to establish a climate where people feel happy with looking for help and sharing their battles. The disgrace encompassing emotional wellness frequently prompts quiet and disconnection, intensifying the difficulties looked by those wrestling with psychological well-being issues.

One of the essential obstructions to tending to psychological well-being concerns is the unavoidable confusions and generalizations that persevere in the public arena. Psychological wellness issues are not an indication of shortcoming or an absence of character; they are intricate circumstances impacted by different variables, including hereditary qualities, science, climate, and valuable encounters. Understanding and sympathy are essential in destroying these confusions and encouraging a climate of empathy and backing.

The effect of psychological well-being on people, families, and networks couldn't possibly be more significant. Psychological wellness issues can appear in different structures, going from state of mind problems like gloom and nervousness to additional serious circumstances like schizophrenia and bipolar issue. The range of emotional well-being difficulties requires a nuanced and far reaching way to deal with care, including counteraction, early intercession, and progressing support.

Prescription For A Healthy Life

Counteraction assumes a significant part in psychological well-being care, underscoring the significance of advancing prosperity and versatility since the beginning. Training and mindfulness projects can assist people with creating survival strategies and stress the executives abilities, lessening the gamble of psychological wellness gives sometime down the road. Establishing strong conditions in schools, work environments, and networks is vital for encouraging capacity to understand anyone on a deeper level and compassion, key parts in keeping up with great psychological well-being.

Early mediation is one more basic part of emotional well-being care. Distinguishing and tending to psychological well-being worries in their beginning phases can forestall the acceleration of issues and work on long haul results. Open and reasonable emotional wellness administrations, combined with destigmatization endeavors, can urge people to look for help unafraid of judgment or segregation.

The job of emotional well-being experts, including specialists, clinicians, advisors, and social laborers, is instrumental in offering the essential help and direction. Nonetheless, the interest for psychological well-being administrations frequently surpasses the accessible assets, featuring the requirement for expanded interest in emotional well-being foundation and labor force advancement. Coordinating psychological well-being into essential consideration settings can improve openness and standardize psychological wellness check-ups as a normal piece of generally speaking medical care.

Notwithstanding proficient help, the job of family and local area can't be put into words. Solid social associations and an emotionally supportive network are defensive variables against psychological wellness challenges. Families, companions, and networks can add to a positive emotional wellness climate by encouraging open correspondence, understanding, and compassion. Building a feeling of local area and lessening social seclusion are fundamental components in making a strong organization for people confronting emotional wellness issues.

The working environment is another basic field where psychological wellness matters. The requests of current workplaces, combined with the tensions of expert life, can add to pressure and psychological wellness challenges. Managers assume an essential part in making work environments that focus on emotional wellness, offering assets and backing to representatives. Adaptable work plans, emotional well-being days, and representative help programs are instances of drives that can add to an intellectually solid work environment culture.

Past the individual and relational levels, cultural factors additionally impact psychological well-being. Financial abberations, separation, and fundamental imbalances can add to the turn of events and worsening of psychological wellness issues. Resolving these more extensive issues requires a complete cultural obligation to equity, value, and inclusivity. Endeavors to destroy foundational hindrances and make an all the more society are naturally connected to advancing emotional well-being for all.

The media and mainstream society likewise assume a huge part in forming view of emotional wellness. Capable and precise depictions of emotional wellness issues in the media can add to diminishing shame and expanding mindfulness. On the other hand, sensationalized or wrong portrayals can propagate destructive generalizations and misinterpretations. Media proficiency and mindful detailing are vital in forming a story that encourages understanding and compassion toward those encountering psychological wellness challenges.

The effect of injury on emotional wellness can't be disregarded. Horrendous encounters, whether coming from youth misfortune, brutality, or different sources, can lastingly affect mental prosperity. Injury informed care accentuates the acknowledgment and comprehension of the effect of injury in offering powerful help and treatment. Making injury informed frameworks across different areas, including medical services, schooling, and law enforcement, is fundamental in tending to the main drivers of emotional well-being difficulties.

Social variety likewise assumes a critical part in understanding and tending to emotional wellness. Various societies might have shifting points of view on emotional wellness, impacting how people see and look for help for psychological well-being issues. Socially able and comprehensive emotional well-being care guarantees that assorted populaces get fitting and compelling help. Perceiving and regarding social contrasts is vital to making an emotional well-being framework that serves everybody evenhandedly.

As social orders advance, so do the difficulties and stressors that influence emotional wellness. Mechanical progressions, virtual entertainment, and the quick moving nature of current life carry the two potential open doors and difficulties to mental prosperity. Adjusting the advantages of innovation with the requirement for disengagement and taking care of oneself is significant in exploring the intricacies of the computerized age. Additionally, tending to the psychological well-being ramifications of arising issues, for example, environmental change and worldwide emergencies, requires creative and versatile methodologies.

Training assumes a vital part in forming perspectives and discernments connected with psychological wellness. Coordinating emotional wellness instruction into school educational programs can furnish youngsters with the information and abilities important to focus on their prosperity and backing others. Instructive foundations likewise have an obligation to establish conditions that advance psychological wellness and prosperity, cultivating a culture of consideration, acknowledgment, and flexibility.

While progress has been made in perceiving the significance of emotional well-being, challenges endure. The worldwide weight of psychological wellness problems keeps on rising, exacerbated by variables like the Coronavirus pandemic, financial shakiness, and international strains. The requirement for an aggregate and composed reaction to psychological well-being has never been more evident.

Legislatures, policymakers, and worldwide associations assume a pivotal part in molding emotional wellness strategies and distributing assets. Focusing on psychological well-being in general wellbeing plans, putting resources into psychological wellness research, and guaranteeing the accessibility of reasonable and available emotional wellness administrations are fundamental stages in tending to the developing emotional wellness emergency. Furthermore, upholding for psychological well-being at the worldwide level adds to the production of a common perspective and obligation to emotional well-being as a worldwide need.

All in all, emotional wellness matters at each degree of society — from the person to the local area, work environment, and then some. It is a crucial part of human prosperity that merits consideration, understanding, and venture. Making an intellectually sound society requires a complex methodology that incorporates counteraction, early mediation, steady conditions, and cultural change. By cooperating to destigmatize psychological wellness, advance mindfulness, and guarantee open and evenhanded consideration, we can construct a reality where psychological wellness genuinely matters for everybody.

5.1 Addressing the importance of mental well-being

Mental prosperity is a foundation of generally wellbeing, impacting people's considerations, feelings, and ways of behaving. As of late, there has been a developing acknowledgment of the significance of mental prosperity as an essential part of a solid and satisfying life. Nonetheless, regardless of expanded mindfulness, psychological wellness challenges continue, and the requirement for a far reaching way to deal with address these issues is more squeezing than any other time.

At its center, mental prosperity envelops close to home versatility, mental well-being, and social agreement. It isn't only the shortfall of mental problems however the presence of positive characteristics like capacity to understand people on a profound level, mindfulness, and the capacity to adapt to life's difficulties.

Mental prosperity is dynamic, impacted by different elements, including hereditary qualities, climate, educational encounters, and cultural standards. Understanding and tending to these elements are pivotal in advancing and keeping up with mental prosperity across assorted populaces.

The disgrace encompassing emotional well-being stays a huge boundary to start discussions and compelling intercessions. Cultural perspectives frequently add to the underestimation of people encountering emotional well-being difficulties, cultivating separation and disengagement. Separating these marks of shame requires an aggregate work to challenge misguided judgments, teach networks, and cultivate sympathy. At the point when people feel happy with examining their psychological prosperity, it makes ready for early intercession and backing.

Counteraction is a vital part of advancing mental prosperity all through the life expectancy. Early mediations that emphasis on building flexibility, adapting abilities, and the capacity to appreciate people on a deeper level can moderate the gamble of emotional well-being issues sometime down the road. Instructive projects pointed toward improving psychological wellness education give people the apparatuses to perceive and address their own psychological prosperity, as well as that of others. By coordinating emotional wellness training into schools and networks, we engage people to play a functioning job in safeguarding their psychological prosperity.

Family and local area support assume an essential part in encouraging mental prosperity. Solid social associations, positive connections, and a steady climate add to close to home strength and a feeling of having a place. Families, as essential social units, can advance mental prosperity by encouraging open correspondence, understanding, and giving a place of refuge to people to communicate their feelings. Networks that focus on friendly attachment and consideration add to the making of conditions that help mental prosperity for everybody.

The work environment is a huge setting where mental prosperity crosses with day to day existence. The requests of present day workplaces, combined with the tensions of expert life, can affect emotional well-being. Managers have an obligation to make work environments that focus on the psychological prosperity of their representatives. This incorporates drives like psychological well-being days, adaptable work game plans, and representative help programs. Developing a steady working environment culture contributes not exclusively to the prosperity of individual representatives yet additionally to by and large efficiency and hierarchical achievement.

Emotional well-being experts, including therapists, clinicians, guides, and social specialists, assume a critical part in supporting people with emotional wellness challenges. Open and reasonable emotional wellness administrations are fundamental for giving ideal mediations and continuous help. Nonetheless, the interest for psychological wellness benefits frequently surpasses accessible assets, featuring the requirement for expanded interest in emotional well-being foundation and labor force advancement.

Incorporating psychological well-being into essential consideration settings can improve openness and standardize emotional well-being check-ups as a normal piece of generally speaking medical services.

Early mediation is basic in tending to emotional well-being difficulties before they raise. Perceiving the indications of mental pain and offering convenient help can forestall the improvement of more serious psychological well-being issues. This requires the accessibility of emotional wellness administrations as well as open mindfulness missions to destigmatize looking for help and support early mediation.

By focusing on psychological wellness in medical services frameworks, we can make a more comprehensive and proactive way to deal with prosperity.

Injury is a critical variable that can influence mental prosperity, frequently appearing as post-horrible pressure problem (PTSD) or other psychological well-being conditions. Injury informed care stresses understanding the impacts of injury and offering help that is delicate to people's previous encounters. Making injury informed frameworks across different areas, including medical services, training, and law enforcement, is fundamental in tending to the underlying drivers of psychological wellness challenges and giving suitable consideration.

Social variety adds one more layer of intricacy to the comprehension and advancement of mental prosperity. Various societies might have differing viewpoints on emotional wellness, impacting how people see and look for help for psychological well-being issues. Social ability in emotional wellness care guarantees that administrations are aware, comprehensive, and compelling for different populaces. Perceiving and regarding social contrasts is vital to making a psychological well-being framework that serves everybody fairly.

Media and mainstream society likewise assume a huge part in forming view of mental prosperity. Mindful and exact depictions of emotional wellness in the media add to lessening disgrace and expanding mindfulness. On the other hand, sensationalized or erroneous portrayals can propagate destructive generalizations and misguided judgments. Media proficiency and mindful revealing are significant in molding a story that cultivates understanding and sympathy toward those encountering psychological wellness challenges.

The effect of financial elements on mental prosperity couldn't possibly be more significant. Neediness, disparity, and absence of admittance to fundamental assets can add to the turn of events and compounding of emotional well-being issues. Tending to these more extensive social determinants of emotional wellness requires an exhaustive cultural obligation to equity, value, and inclusivity. Endeavors to destroy fundamental obstructions and make an all the more society are naturally connected to advancing mental prosperity for all.

As social orders develop, new difficulties and stressors arise that can affect mental prosperity. The computerized age, set apart by innovative progressions and the pervasiveness of web-based entertainment, acquaints the two open doors and difficulties with mental prosperity. Adjusting the advantages of innovation with the requirement for disengagement and taking care of oneself is critical in exploring the intricacies of the advanced time. Besides, tending to the psychological well-being ramifications of arising issues, for example, environmental change and worldwide emergencies, requires creative and versatile methodologies.

Schooling assumes a vital part in molding perspectives and discernments connected with mental prosperity. Coordinating psychological wellness instruction into school educational plans furnishes youngsters with the information and abilities important to focus on their prosperity and backing others. Instructive foundations likewise have an obligation to establish conditions that advance mental prosperity, cultivating a culture of thoughtfulness, acknowledgment, and strength.

While progress has been made in perceiving the significance of mental prosperity, challenges persevere. The worldwide weight of emotional wellness problems keeps on rising, exacerbated by variables like the Coronavirus pandemic, monetary unsteadiness, and international pressures. The requirement for an aggregate and composed reaction to mental prosperity has never been more obvious.

Legislatures, policymakers, and worldwide associations assume a vital part in molding strategies that focus on mental prosperity. Designating assets to emotional well-being research, guaranteeing the accessibility of reasonable and available emotional well-being administrations, and destigmatizing looking for help are fundamental stages in tending to the developing emotional wellness emergency. Furthermore, upholding for mental prosperity at the worldwide level adds to the making of a mutual perspective and obligation to psychological wellness as a key part of common freedoms.

All in all, tending to the significance of mental prosperity requires a multilayered and cooperative methodology. From counteraction and early intercession to establishing strong conditions and tending to foundational imbalances, advancing mental prosperity is a common obligation. By cultivating open discussions, testing marks of shame, and focusing on emotional well-being in all parts of life, we can construct a general public where mental prosperity isn't recently perceived however effectively supported and safeguarded.

5.2 Discussing stress management techniques

Stress is an unavoidable piece of life, influencing people in different ways and at various forces. Whether it's connected with work, connections, monetary worries, or other life pressures, finding compelling pressure the board methods is fundamental for keeping up with by and large prosperity. In the present high speed and requesting world, the capacity to adapt to pressure is an important expertise that can essentially influence mental and actual wellbeing.

This conversation will investigate a scope of stress the executives procedures, incorporating both proactive ways to deal with forestall pressure and receptive systems to adapt to it when it emerges.

Proactive Pressure The board Methods:

Care and Contemplation:

Care rehearses include developing consciousness of the current second without judgment. Contemplation, a critical part of care, empowers centered consideration and unwinding. Methods like profound breathing, directed symbolism, and moderate muscle unwinding fall under this class. Standard care and reflection can upgrade mindfulness, lessen uneasiness, and work on generally speaking mental versatility.

Normal Activity:

Active work is a strong pressure minimizer. Practice discharges endorphins, the body's regular state of mind lifters, and gives an outlet to gathered pressure. Whether it's a lively walk, a rec center exercise, or taking part in a most loved sport, integrating customary activity into one's standard adds to both physical and mental prosperity.

Solid Way of life Decisions:

Sustenance, rest, and hydration assume urgent parts in pressure the board. An even eating regimen gives the body fundamental supplements, supporting ideal working. Satisfactory rest is fundamental for mental capability and close to home guideline. Hydration is likewise connected to mental execution and can impact temperament. Focusing on a sound way of life sets a strong starting point for overseeing pressure.

Using time productively:

Powerful using time effectively can diminish sensations of being overpowered. Breaking errands into more modest, reasonable advances, focusing on liabilities, and laying out practical objectives add to a feeling of control. Time usage procedures, for example, the Pomodoro Method or the Eisenhower Framework, assist people with designating their time effectively and keep away from the unfavorable impacts of hesitation.

Social Associations:

Keeping up areas of strength for with associations offers profound help during testing times. Conversing with companions, family, or partners about stressors can offer alternate points of view and survival techniques. Mingling and participating in charming exercises with others cultivate a feeling of having a place and lessen sensations of separation.

Defining Limits:

Laying out clear limits in private and expert life is significant for forestalling burnout and persistent pressure. Figuring out how to say no while important, focusing on taking care of oneself, and imparting individual cutoff points are fundamental parts of defining and keeping up with sound limits.

Responsive Pressure The board Procedures:

Mental Social Methods:

Mental Social Treatment (CBT) is a broadly perceived approach for overseeing pressure. It includes distinguishing and testing negative idea examples and supplanting them with additional productive ones. CBT strategies, for example, reexamining, can assist people with acquiring a superior viewpoint on stressors and foster better approaches to adapting.

Expressive Composition:

Expounding on one's viewpoints and feelings, known as expressive composition, can be a therapeutic and stress-easing movement. Journaling gives an outlet to self-articulation and reflection, helping people cycle and get a handle on their sentiments in the midst of stress.

Moderate Muscle Unwinding (PMR):

PMR is an unwinding strategy that includes straining and afterward bit by bit delivering different muscle bunches in the body. This cycle advances actual unwinding and can assist with easing the muscle pressure frequently connected with pressure. Normal act of PMR can add to by and large pressure decrease.

Biofeedback and Unwinding Applications:

Biofeedback includes observing physiological signs, for example, pulse or muscle pressure, and figuring out how to control them for stress decrease. In the advanced age, different unwinding applications and wearable gadgets offer biofeedback elements to assist people with overseeing pressure continuously. These apparatuses frequently incorporate directed contemplations, breathing activities, and stress following functionalities.

Critical thinking Procedures:

Recognizing the underlying drivers of stress and creating successful critical thinking methodologies can address stressors straightforwardly. This approach includes separating difficulties into sensible advances, looking for help when required, and going to proactive lengths to forestall comparable stressors later on.

Workmanship and Inventiveness:

Participating in imaginative exercises, whether it's painting, drawing, composing, or playing an instrument, gives a remedial outlet to self-articulation. Imaginative undertakings can be a type of care, permitting people to zero in on the inventive strategy and briefly shift their consideration away from stressors.

Mind-Body Mediations:

Rehearses that incorporate the brain and body, like yoga and kendo, are powerful pressure the board procedures. These disciplines consolidate actual development, breath control, and care to advance unwinding and balance. Customary cooperation at the top of the priority list body mediations can work on generally speaking flexibility to stretch.

Proficient Help:

Looking for the direction of psychological well-being experts, like advisors or advocates, can be fundamental for overseeing constant or overpowering pressure. These experts can give customized procedures, methods for dealing with especially difficult times, and a place of refuge for people to investigate and address the hidden reasons for their pressure.

Consolidating Techniques for All encompassing Pressure The executives:

Successfully overseeing pressure frequently includes a blend of proactive and receptive systems. Fostering a customized tool compartment of stress the board strategies permits people to pick the most proper methodology in light of the particular stressors they experience. Coordinating sound way of life decisions, cultivating social associations, and integrating unwinding rehearses into everyday schedules add to an all encompassing way to deal with pressure the executives.

It's essential to perceive that the adequacy of stress the board methods can differ from one individual to another. What functions admirably for one individual may not be as successful for another. Trying different things with various methodologies and focusing on individual inclinations and reactions is critical to tracking down a customized and feasible way to deal with pressure the board.

All in all, stress is an omnipresent part of life, yet what people answer and oversee pressure fundamentally means for their general prosperity. Proactive methodologies, like care, work out, and sound way of life decisions, add to versatility and forestall the adverse consequence of stress. Responsive procedures, including mental social methodologies, expressive composition, and unwinding rehearses, offer devices for adapting to pressure when it emerges. By consolidating different pressure the executives procedures and fitting them to individual necessities, people can develop a reasonable and versatile way to deal with exploring life's difficulties.

5.3 Exploring mindfulness and meditation practices

Care and reflection rehearses have earned inescapable respect as integral assets for advancing mental prosperity, lessening pressure, and upgrading by and large personal satisfaction. Established in old pondering customs, these practices have found a spot in contemporary society as proof based ways to deal with dealing with the intricacies of present day life. This investigation dives into the ideas of care and reflection, their authentic roots, the science behind their adequacy, and commonsense applications in day to day existence.

Figuring out Care:

At its center, care includes developing an increased consciousness of the current second with a demeanor of non-judgment. This mindfulness envelops one's considerations, feelings, and actual sensations. Instead of choosing not to move on or stressing over the future, care urges people to draw in with the ongoing experience completely.

Care isn't tied in with disposing of contemplations however noticing them without connection, considering an additional fair and objective point of view.

Authentic Underlying foundations of Care:

Care has its starting points in antiquated thoughtful practices, especially in Buddhist customs. The expression "care" is frequently interpreted from the Pali word "sati" or the Sanskrit word "smṛti," the two of which allude to the development of mindfulness and consideration. In Buddhist way of thinking, care is a fundamental part of the Eightfold Way, a manual for moral and mental turn of events.

Thich Nhat Hanh, a Vietnamese Harmony Buddhist priest, is credited with promoting care in the West. His lessons underline the reconciliation of care into day to day existence, changing routine exercises into open doors for mindfulness and presence. The boundless reception of care based intercessions, for example, Care Based Pressure Decrease (MBSR) and Care Based Mental Treatment (MBCT), has added to the reconciliation of care into standard psychological wellness rehearses.

The Study of Care:

Logical examination has given indisputable proof to the beneficial outcomes of care on mental and actual prosperity. Neuroscientific concentrates on utilizing cerebrum imaging methods, for example, useful attractive reverberation imaging (fMRI), have shown underlying changes in the mind related with care practice. The regions engaged with consideration, profound guideline, and mindfulness exhibit expanded action and network.

One prominent cerebrum locale embroiled in care is the prefrontal cortex, liable for chief capabilities, for example, navigation and drive control. Care rehearses have been related with changes in the amygdala, a vital locale in the cerebrum's close to home handling. These neurobiological changes recommend that care might add to worked on profound guideline and flexibility.

The act of care has been connected to decreases in apparent pressure and side effects of tension and wretchedness. Studies have demonstrated the way that standard care practice can prompt changes in the autonomic sensory system, bringing about diminished physiological markers of stress, for example, cortisol levels and pulse. Also, care based intercessions have been incorporated into clinical settings to help people managing different emotional wellness challenges.

Key Parts of Care Practices:

Centered Consideration (Fixation):

Care frequently starts with creating centered consideration. This includes guiding one's attention to a particular mark of concentration, like the breath, a mantra, or a specific sensation. The point is to develop supported consideration and fixation, preparing the psyche to remain present without becoming entrapped in interruptions.

Non-Critical Mindfulness:

Fundamental to care is the act of non-critical mindfulness. This includes noticing considerations and feelings without appending names of positive or negative. Instead of responding indiscreetly to interior encounters, people figure out how to answer with serenity and acknowledgment. This non-critical position cultivates a caring relationship with one's own considerations and feelings.

Body Sweep:

The body check is a care practice that includes deliberately focusing on various pieces of the body. This assists people with fostering an elevated consciousness of substantial sensations, advancing an association between the psyche and body. The body examine is normally utilized in care based mediations to improve present-second mindfulness.

Prescription For A Healthy Life

Careful Relaxing:
Careful breathing, or careful familiarity with the breath, is an essential practice in numerous care customs. By zeroing in consideration on the breath, people can moor themselves right now. The breath fills in as a perspective, offering a promptly accessible and consistent anchor for developing care.

Open Observing:
Open checking includes noticing one's contemplations and feelings without obsession with a particular mark of concentration. Rather than focusing on a specific item, people keep an open familiarity with the whole area of involvement. This type of care energizes an extensive and open mindfulness, considering a complete comprehension of the brain's exercises.

Useful Utilizations of Care:

Stress Decrease:
Care is broadly perceived for its pressure decreasing impacts. By encouraging an attention to the current second, people can interfere with the pattern of stressors and responses. Care rehearses, for example, profound breathing and body check, give apparatuses to overseeing pressure continuously. Ordinary care practice has been related with lower seen feelings of anxiety and expanded flexibility notwithstanding challenges.

Profound Guideline:
Care improves close to home guideline by advancing a non-responsive familiarity with feelings. Instead of being overpowered or constrained by feelings, people can notice them with separation. This takes into consideration a more deliberate and thought about reaction to close to home encounters, adding to profound prosperity.

Further developed Focus and Mental Working:
The development of centered consideration in care rehearses adds to further developed fixation and mental working. Research recommends that normal care practice can upgrade working memory, mental adaptability, and generally speaking mental execution.

These advantages reach out past conventional reflection meetings to everyday assignments that require supported consideration.

Upgraded Mindfulness:
Care develops mindfulness by empowering people to investigate their inward encounters without judgment. This uplifted mindfulness reaches out to contemplations, feelings, and substantial sensations. By turning out to be more sensitive to their inside scene, people can pursue informed decisions lined up with their qualities and objectives.

Careful Eating:
Care can be applied to day to day exercises, including eating. Careful eating includes giving full consideration to the tangible experience of eating, enjoying

each chomp, and being sensitive to craving and completion signs. This training advances a better relationship with food, forestalling careless eating and encouraging a more cognizant way to deal with nourishment.

Rest Improvement:

Rest cleanliness is vital for generally speaking prosperity, and care practices can add to further developed rest. Care based mediations, for example, care based a sleeping disorder treatment (MBIT), have shown guarantee in tending to rest unsettling influences. By advancing unwinding and lessening pre-rest mental excitement, care can add to all the more likely rest quality.

Investigating Reflection Practices:

Reflection, frequently entwined with care, envelops a different exhibit of scrutinizing rehearses pointed toward developing mental clearness, close to home equilibrium, and otherworldly knowledge. While care can be viewed as a type of contemplation, reflection rehearses stretch out past the mindfulness centered procedures examined before. How about we dig into some key contemplation rehearses, their verifiable roots, and their contemporary applications.

Authentic Foundations of Reflection:

The act of contemplation has profound authentic roots, crossing different societies and otherworldly customs. In Eastern customs, contemplation has been an essential piece of Hinduism and Buddhism for quite a long time. The old text, the Bhagavad Gita, portrays contemplation as a way to self-acknowledgment and association with the heavenly. In Buddhism, contemplation is vital to the Eightfold Way, directing specialists toward freedom from misery.

Contemplation is a training that has been embraced by different societies and customs for a really long time. It is a strategy for preparing the psyche to accomplish a condition of mental lucidity, concentration, and unwinding. The starting points of contemplation can be followed back to old developments, where it was frequently connected with otherworldly and strict practices. After some time, contemplation has developed and taken on different structures, each with its own procedures and purposes.

One of the most notable types of contemplation is care reflection. This training has its foundations in Buddhist practices yet has acquired broad prevalence in mainstream settings. Care reflection includes focusing on the current second without judgment. Experts frequently center around their breath, substantial sensations, or the climate around them. The objective is to develop mindfulness and foster a non-receptive, tolerating mentality.

One more generally rehearsed type of reflection is supernatural contemplation (TM). TM is a mantra-based reflection strategy that was presented by Maharishi Mahesh Yogi during the 1950s. During TM, people rehash a particular mantra quietly to themselves, permitting the psyche to sink into a condition of profound peaceful mindfulness. The training is intended to advance unwinding and lessen pressure, at last prompting expanded unwavering focus and worked on in general prosperity.

Directed reflection is a type of contemplation where people adhere to the guidelines of an aide, either face to face or through sound accounts. This sort of contemplation is frequently utilized for unwinding, stress decrease, and self-awareness. The aide might lead members through perceptions, body examines, or centered consideration works out. Directed contemplation can be particularly useful for novices who might find it trying to reflect without outside direction.

Adoring graciousness contemplation, or metta reflection, is established in Buddhist practices and spotlights on developing sensations of adoration and sympathy towards oneself as well as other people. Experts normally rehash expressions or assertions that express generosity and benevolence. This type of reflection means to cultivate a feeling of association, compassion, and good feelings.

Chakra contemplation is a training that includes adjusting and adjusting the body's energy habitats, known as chakras. In Hindu and yogic practices, it is accepted that the body has seven principal chakras, each related with explicit characteristics and feelings. Chakra reflection includes picturing or focusing on each chakra to advance equilibrium and congruity in both the physical and enthusiastic parts of oneself.

Development based contemplation rehearses, like kendo and qigong, coordinate actual development with care and breath mindfulness. These practices began in Chinese combative techniques and are frequently portrayed as "contemplation moving." The sluggish, purposeful developments expect to advance unwinding, balance, and the progression of essential energy all through the body.

Harmony contemplation, or zazen, is a type of situated reflection that is fundamental to Harmony Buddhism. During zazen, experts sit in a particular stance, frequently on a pad, zeroing in on their breath and noticing considerations without connection. The objective is to encounter direct understanding into the idea of the real world and achieve a condition of profound mindfulness and presence.

Yoga nidra, otherwise called yogic rest, is a type of directed contemplation that incites a condition of cognizant unwinding. Members rests in an agreeable situation while an aide leads them through an efficient course of body mindfulness and profound unwinding. The training is intended to advance physical, mental, and profound unwinding while at the same time keeping a condition of cognizant mindfulness.

Supernatural Contemplation, or TM, is a generally polished type of mantra reflection. Presented by Maharishi Mahesh Yogi during the 1950s, TM includes the quiet redundancy of a particular mantra to accomplish a condition of profound peaceful mindfulness. The training expects to advance unwinding, lessen pressure, and upgrade by and large prosperity.

Care Based Pressure Decrease (MBSR) is an organized program that joins care reflection and yoga to lessen pressure and improve prosperity. Created by Dr. Jon Kabat-Zinn in the last part of the 1970s, MBSR has been generally taken on in clinical settings as a corresponding way to deal with overseeing different medical issue, including persistent torment and nervousness.

Notwithstanding these particular contemplation rehearses, there are incalculable varieties and blends that people can investigate to find what impacts them actually. The ongoing idea among these practices is the development of an increased condition of mindfulness, center, and inward harmony.

No matter what the particular type of reflection, professionals frequently experience a scope of advantages that stretch out past the contemplation meeting itself. Research has demonstrated the way that customary reflection practice can add to worked on mental and actual prosperity. A portion of the key advantages incorporate diminished pressure, upgraded close to home guideline, expanded consideration and fixation, and further developed rest quality.

Stress decrease is one of the most broadly perceived advantages of reflection. In the present quick moving world, many individuals experience constant pressure, which can add to an assortment of medical problems. Reflection gives an instrument to balance the impacts of pressure by advancing unwinding and enacting the body's normal unwinding reaction.

One of the manners in which contemplation decreases pressure is by directing the body's pressure chemical, cortisol. At the point when the body is in a condition of persistent pressure, cortisol levels can become raised, prompting a scope of negative wellbeing impacts. Ordinary contemplation has been displayed to bring down cortisol levels, assisting people with overseeing pressure all the more actually.

Past pressure decrease, contemplation has been connected to enhancements in close to home prosperity. The act of care, specifically, urges people to notice their contemplations and feelings without judgment. This non-receptive mindfulness can prompt more prominent close to home flexibility and an additional reasonable point of view on life's difficulties.

Studies have additionally found that reflection can emphatically influence consideration and mental capability. The engaged consideration expected during reflection practices can improve fixation and mental control. This is reflected in research showing enhancements in assignments connected with consideration, memory, and critical thinking among normal meditators.

The advantages of contemplation are not restricted to the psychological domain; there are likewise eminent actual impacts. Contemplation has been related with changes in mind construction and capability. For instance, neuroimaging studies have shown modifications in the size and movement of cerebrum locales engaged with consideration, mindfulness, and profound guideline.

Prescription For A Healthy Life

Additionally, contemplation has been connected to enhancements in rest quality. Numerous people battle with rest unsettling influences, and exploration recommends that contemplation can be an important device for advancing better rest. Practices, for example, care reflection and yoga nidra, with their emphasis on unwinding and body mindfulness, can be particularly powerful in further developing rest designs.

Notwithstanding these general advantages, different reflection practices might offer exceptional benefits. For instance, adoring benevolence reflection has been related with expanded sensations of empathy and social connectedness. Chakra contemplation might add to a feeling of equilibrium and essentialness by tending to the vivacious parts of the body. Development based rehearses like yoga and qigong advance actual wellbeing as well as develop care through facilitated development and breath.

Notwithstanding the boundless advantages, moving toward contemplation with practical expectations is fundamental. While certain individuals might encounter prompt beneficial outcomes, others might demand greater investment to see changes. Consistency is critical, as the combined effect of ordinary practice will in general enhance the advantages after some time.

Beginning with reflection requires no exceptional gear or skill. Amateurs can investigate different contemplation styles to find what impacts them. Here are a down to earth moves toward start a reflection practice:

Pick an Agreeable Stance: Whether sitting or resting, find an agreeable place that permits you to be ready and loose. If sitting, keep a straight spine to help mindful mindfulness.

Select a Calm Climate: Pick a peaceful space where you will not be quickly upset. Quietness your telephone and establish a climate helpful for center.

Set a Reasonable Length: Begin with a sensible term, like 5 to 10 minutes, and step by step increment it as you become more acclimated with the training.

Center around the Breath: Numerous contemplation rehearses include focusing on the breath. Notice the impression of each breathe in and breathe out, and tenderly take your consideration back to the breath assuming that your brain meanders.

Be Patient and Non-Critical: It's normal for the brain to meander during reflection. Rather than becoming disappointed, essentially recognize the interruption and tenderly aide your concentration back to the current second.

Explore different avenues regarding Various Styles: Investigate different reflection styles to find what impacts you. Whether it's care, cherishing thoughtfulness, or development based rehearses, there's a large number of choices to suit various inclinations.

Think about Directed Contemplations: In the event that you're new to reflection, directed meetings drove by experienced teachers can give design and backing. Numerous applications and online stages offer directed reflection accounts.

Lay out a Daily schedule: Consistency is significant in building a reflection practice. Put away a particular time every day to develop the propensity.

Be Available to Encounters: Contemplation is an individual excursion, and encounters can shift. Be available to the various sensations, considerations, and feelings that might emerge during your training.

Chapter 6

Sleep for Vitality

Rest is a basic part of human life, a physiological need that assumes a urgent part in keeping up with generally speaking wellbeing and prosperity. While the significance of rest is generally recognized, its importance frequently will in general be disregarded or misjudged in our high speed, current lives. Chasing after efficiency and achievement, numerous people penance valuable long periods of rest, uninformed about the significant effect this can have on their physical and emotional wellness.

The idea of "rest for imperativeness" underscores the significant job that satisfactory and quality rest plays in advancing essentialness - a condition of hearty wellbeing, energy, and strength. In this investigation of rest and essentialness, we dig into the unpredictable components of rest, disentangle the outcomes of lack of sleep, and divulge the heap manners by which focusing on rest can upgrade our imperativeness.

At its center, rest is a mind boggling and dynamic cycle that unfurls in different stages, each serving extraordinary capabilities. The rest cycle comprises of two principal classes: quick eye development (REM) rest and non-fast eye development (NREM) rest. NREM rest is additionally partitioned into three phases, with each stage set apart by particular physiological changes. As people progress through these stages throughout the span of the evening, the body goes through cycles of reclamation, memory combination, and close to home guideline.

During NREM rest, the body participates in fix and upkeep exercises. Tissues are recovered, energy is reestablished, and the safe framework reinforces its guards. This stage is fundamental for actual recuperation, as development chemical is delivered, adding to the maintenance of muscles and tissues. The body additionally directs different metabolic cycles during NREM rest, affecting variables, for example, glucose levels and hunger.

Interestingly, REM rest is portrayed by quick eye developments, expanded mind action, and distinctive dreaming. REM rest is especially essential for mental capabilities and close to home prosperity. It is during this stage that the cerebrum solidifies recollections, processes feelings, and participates in imaginative critical thinking. Denying oneself of REM rest can prompt hindered mental capability, memory deficiencies, and profound shakiness.

The results of lack of sleep are significant and expansive. Past the prompt sensations of weakness and touchiness, persistent lack of sleep can have extreme ramifications for both physical and psychological wellness. According to a physiological point of view, deficient rest is related with an expanded gamble of cardiovascular illnesses, diabetes, and weight. The insusceptible framework likewise debilitates, delivering the body more powerless to diseases.

Intellectually, the impacts of lack of sleep are striking. Hindered fixation, decreased critical thinking skills, and a decrease in generally speaking mental execution are normal results. Additionally, ongoing lack of sleep has been connected to a raised gamble of neurodegenerative circumstances like Alzheimer's infection. The mind boggling connection among rest and cerebrum wellbeing highlights the significance of focusing on rest for mental essentialness.

Inwardly, rest assumes a urgent part in controlling temperament and overseeing pressure. Lack of sleep can prompt elevated profound reactivity, expanded crabbiness, and a more noteworthy helplessness to mind-set problems like tension and misery. The unpredictable exchange among rest and profound prosperity highlights the significance of integrating adequate rest into one's daily practice as an essential part of emotional well-being upkeep.

In the domain of efficiency and execution, the effect of rest is unquestionable. In opposition to the conviction that forfeiting rest for additional functioning hours improves efficiency, research reliably exhibits that sleepless people are not so much productive but rather more inclined to mistakes. Also, the capacity to enhance, issue address, and think innovatively is compromised when the cerebrum is denied of the supportive impacts of rest.

The cultural standards and assumptions that frequently commend hecticness and lack of sleep add to a culture where people might disregard their rest needs for work or social responsibilities. The idea of working really hard as an image of commitment and achievement has profound social roots, propagating a mentality that values efficiency over prosperity. Nonetheless, a change in perspective is fundamental, perceiving that genuine imperativeness and achievement originate from an all encompassing methodology that focuses on both expert accomplishment and individual wellbeing.

The connection among rest and essentialness stretches out past the physical and mental domains; it significantly impacts relational connections and social elements. Lack of sleep can prompt uplifted crabbiness, hindered relational abilities, and a diminished capacity to identify with others. Thusly, the nature of connections, both individual and expert, may endure when people are constantly restless.

Nurturing, specifically, uncovers the difficulties of adjusting rest and providing care liabilities. Restless evenings with babies and small kids are a transitional experience for some guardians, yet the drawn out effect of persistent lack of sleep on parental prosperity and the parent-youngster relationship is a subject of developing concern. Perceiving the significance of parental rest for the general relational intricacy is fundamental for encouraging a solid and sustaining climate.

The unavoidable impact of innovation in contemporary society has acquainted new difficulties with accomplishing relaxing and helpful rest. The commonness of screens in our regular routines, from cell phones to PCs, has been connected to disturbances in rest designs. The blue light transmitted by screens can obstruct the creation of melatonin, a chemical that directs rest wake cycles, making it more challenging to nod off.

Also, the consistent network worked with by innovation has obscured the limits among work and individual life. The assumption for being reachable at painfully inconvenient times can add to elevated feelings of anxiety and disturb the regular cadence of rest. Laying out solid limits with innovation, for example, carrying out computerized curfews and making an innovation free sleep time schedule, is significant for recovering soothing rest in the computerized age.

Establishing an ideal rest climate is one more key figure upgrading the nature of rest. Factors like room temperature, lighting, and clamor levels can fundamentally affect rest quality. A cool, dim, and calm climate is helpful for tranquil rest, advancing the body's normal circadian musicality. Putting resources into an agreeable bedding and cushions that offer legitimate help is likewise fundamental for making a rest shelter that advances imperativeness.

The significance of rest cleanliness, including propensities and practices that advance sound rest, couldn't possibly be more significant. Laying out a reliable rest plan, keeping an unwinding pre-rest schedule, and keeping away from energizers, for example, caffeine and nicotine near sleep time add to the general nature of rest.

Developing care and stress-diminishing practices, like reflection and profound breathing activities, can additionally improve the capacity to loosen up and set up the psyche for tranquil rest.

Perceiving the singular changeability in rest needs is fundamental in the mission for essentialness. While the suggested term of rest for grown-ups is by and large between 7 to 9 hours out of every evening, individual prerequisites might shift. Factors like age, hereditary qualities, and generally speaking wellbeing impact the ideal measure of rest required for every individual. Paying attention to one's body and focusing on rest as indicated by individual requirements is an essential move toward accomplishing and keeping up with imperativeness.

The quest for imperativeness through rest isn't bound to evening time hours alone; the idea stretches out to the significance of snoozing as an essential device for upgrading daytime readiness and execution. Short rests, regularly enduring between 10 to 30 minutes, can give a fast jolt of energy without the sluggishness related with longer rests. Snoozing in a calculated way, like in the early evening, lines up with the body's normal circadian musicality and can be a significant part of a balanced way to deal with rest for imperativeness.

In working environments that focus on representative prosperity, the acknowledgment of the connection among rest and efficiency has prompted the execution of drives, for example, adaptable work hours and assigned rest spaces. Recognizing that very much refreshed representatives are more drawn in, imaginative, and versatile, associations are progressively perceiving the significance of cultivating a culture that welcomes rests.

6.1 Highlighting the importance of quality sleep

Quality rest is a fundamental part of in general prosperity, affecting different parts of physical and emotional well-being. In our speedy current culture, where efficiency and steady network are exceptionally esteemed, the significance of value rest is frequently underrated. This oversight can prompt a horde of medical problems and adversely influence mental capability, close to home prosperity, and even life span.

The meaning of value rest stretches out past the ordinarily known advantages of feeling refreshed and alert. It assumes a vital part in keeping a sound resistant framework, directing chemicals, and supporting legitimate mind capability. In this complete investigation, we will dig into the diverse parts of rest, disentangling the science behind it, grasping its effect on various aspects of life, and investigating methodologies to upgrade rest quality.

Deductively, rest is a complex physiological interaction that includes various stages and cycles. The two principal kinds of rest are fast eye development (REM) rest and non-REM rest. Non-REM rest comprises of three phases, each serving explicit capabilities like actual rebuilding and memory union. REM rest, then again, is related with distinctive dreaming and mental rebuilding.

During rest, the body goes through different cycles that are essential for keeping up with ideal wellbeing. One of the essential elements of rest is to permit the body to fix and recover tissues. This incorporates the maintenance of muscles, bones, and different cells that might have been harmed during everyday exercises. Also, rest is fundamental for the legitimate working of the insusceptible framework.

The safe framework is a mind boggling organization of cells and proteins that shield the body against destructive trespassers, like microbes and infections. Quality rest is firmly connected to resistant capability, and inadequate or low quality rest can debilitate the insusceptible reaction. Persistent lack of sleep has been related with an expanded helplessness to diseases, making people more inclined to sicknesses.

Besides, rest assumes a vital part in the guideline of chemicals that are fundamental for different physical processes. Chemicals like development chemical, cortisol, insulin, and melatonin follow a circadian mood, which is impacted by the rest wake cycle. Disturbances in this cycle, frequently brought about by unpredictable rest examples or rest problems, can prompt hormonal uneven characters, adding to a scope of medical problems.

One chemical intently attached to rest is melatonin, frequently alluded to as the "rest chemical." Melatonin is created by the pineal organ in light of dimness and manages the rest wake cycle. Openness to fake light, particularly from electronic gadgets, can smother melatonin creation, disturbing the normal rest wake mood and making it trying to nod off.

The effect of rest on mental capability is significant. Memory union, learning, and critical abilities to think are altogether impacted by the quality and amount of rest. During the different rest arranges, the cerebrum processes and combines data procured over the course of the day. Deficient rest can debilitate mental capability, prompting challenges in fixation, memory review, and direction.

The connection among rest and psychological wellness is unpredictable, with rest unsettling influences frequently connected to state of mind problems, tension, and despondency. Ongoing lack of sleep can worsen existing psychological wellness conditions and add to the advancement of new ones. The bidirectional idea of this relationship stresses the significance of tending to rest as a principal part of psychological well-being care.

Stress, a pervasive part of current life, can both upset rest and be exacerbated by unfortunate rest. The body's pressure reaction, intervened by the arrival of cortisol, is complicatedly associated with the rest wake cycle. Persistent pressure can prompt hyperarousal, making it hard for people to unwind and nod off. On the other hand, absence of rest can increment feelings of anxiety, making a cycle that adversely influences both physical and mental prosperity.

Notwithstanding the physiological viewpoints, the cultural and way of life factors affecting rest can't be disregarded. The approach of innovation and the every minute of every day accessibility of data have obscured the limits among work and individual life, frequently infringing on valuable rest time. The commonness of cell phones, tablets, and workstations has presented a consistent stream of notices, adding to rest unsettling influences and diminished rest quality.

Shift work, a typical element in numerous ventures, represents a critical test to keeping a normal rest plan. The disturbance of the normal circadian musicality can prompt rest problems, weakness, and long haul wellbeing results. Night shift laborers, specifically, face an expanded gamble of different medical problems, including cardiovascular sicknesses and metabolic issues.

The significance of value rest reaches out to actual wellbeing, with rest assuming an essential part in weight the board and digestion. Lack of sleep has been related with an expanded gamble of weight, insulin obstruction, and type 2 diabetes. Disturbances in the rest wake cycle can influence hunger-controlling chemicals, prompting an awkwardness in craving and possibly adding to gorging.

The connection among rest and cardiovascular wellbeing is deeply grounded. Constant lack of sleep has been connected to an expanded gamble of hypertension, coronary conduit sickness, and stroke. Rest problems like rest apnea, portrayed by breaks in breathing during rest, further raise the gamble of cardiovascular issues. Perceiving the exchange among rest and cardiovascular wellbeing highlights the significance of focusing on quality rest for by and large prosperity.

The effect of rest on life span is a subject of expanding interest in logical exploration. Concentrates reliably show a relationship between adequate, great rest and expanded future. On the other hand, constant lack of sleep has been connected to a higher mortality risk. Understanding the job of stay in bed advancing life span stresses its importance as a crucial mainstay of a sound way of life.

The nature of rest not set in stone by the span spent in bed yet additionally by the consistency and profundity of the rest stages. Rest problems, like a sleeping disorder, rest apnea, and a propensity to fidget, can fundamentally think twice about quality. Tending to these problems is fundamental for guaranteeing supportive rest and receiving the full rewards of the rest interaction.

The effect of innovation on rest quality is a developing worry in contemporary society. The boundless utilization of electronic gadgets, especially at night, opens people to fake light that can slow down the creation of melatonin, making it trying to start rest.

The habit-forming nature of virtual entertainment and online substance further adds to deferred sleep times and divided rest.

Establishing a rest helpful climate is central for improving rest quality. The room ought to be a safe-haven committed to rest and unwinding. This includes limiting clamor, guaranteeing an agreeable sleeping cushion and pads, and controlling the room's temperature. Furthermore, the utilization of power outage draperies can assist with establishing an ideal rest climate by shutting out outside light.

Laying out a reliable rest routine is a vital procedure for further developing rest quality. Heading to sleep and awakening simultaneously consistently manages the body's inside clock, building up the normal circadian musicality. Keeping away from caffeine and invigorating exercises near sleep time, as well as restricting openness to screens, upholds the change into a tranquil state.

The connection among diet and rest is unpredictable, with healthful decisions affecting rest quality. Certain food sources contain intensifies that can either advance or thwart rest. For instance, food sources wealthy in tryptophan, like turkey and dairy items, can add to the creation of serotonin and melatonin, advancing unwinding and rest. Then again, consuming energizers like caffeine near sleep time can upset rest.

Customary active work has been reliably connected to further developed rest quality. Participating in moderate-power work out, like strolling or cycling, can advance serene rest. In any case, it is crucial for time active work suitably, keeping away from enthusiastic activity near sleep time, as this might make an invigorating difference. The connection among exercise and rest highlights the all encompassing methodology expected for ideal prosperity.

Mind-body rehearses, like contemplation and unwinding procedures, can be compelling in advancing rest quality. These practices assist with quieting the brain and decrease pressure, establishing a helpful climate for peaceful rest. Integrating care into the sleep time routine can flag the body to progress into a condition of unwinding, working with the beginning of rest.

Mental social treatment for sleep deprivation (CBT-I) has arisen as an exceptionally successful, proof based approach for tending to rest problems. CBT-I centers around distinguishing and changing contemplations and ways of behaving that add to a sleeping disorder. This helpful methodology intends to further develop rest cleanliness, lay out a predictable rest schedule, and address negative idea designs connected with rest.

The job of pharmacological mediations, for example, rest prescriptions, in overseeing rest issues ought to be drawn nearer carefully. While these prescriptions might give momentary help, they accompany likely aftereffects and the gamble of reliance. Interview with a medical services proficient is vital while considering pharmacological mediations for rest issues, and their utilization ought to be essential for a thorough therapy plan.

Perceiving the effect of rest on psychological well-being, working environments are progressively focusing on representative prosperity by carrying out approaches that help sound rest propensities. Adaptable plans for getting work done, assigned rest regions, and mindfulness programs on the significance of rest add to encouraging a rest well disposed workplace. Businesses assume a significant part in advancing a sound balance between serious and fun activities, recognizing that sufficient rest is essential to worker execution and fulfillment.

Teaching general society about the significance of value rest is fundamental for encouraging a culture that values rest and focuses on prosperity. General wellbeing efforts can bring issues to light about the outcomes of constant lack of sleep and give data on sound rest propensities. Schools and work environments can likewise assume a part in advancing rest training, stressing its effect on scholar and word related execution.

The job of medical care experts in tending to rest related issues is principal. Essential consideration suppliers can assume a critical part in recognizing and overseeing rest issues, leading exhaustive evaluations, and working together with experts when fundamental. Coordinating rest evaluations into routine medical care visits can assist with distinguishing potential issues from the get-go, forestalling the acceleration of rest related issues.

The significance of value rest stretches out to weak populaces, like kids and the older. Youngsters, specifically, require adequate rest for development, improvement, and scholastic achievement. Laying out solid rest propensities since the beginning sets the establishment for deep rooted prosperity. Additionally, more seasoned grown-ups may confront extraordinary difficulties connected with rest, remembering changes for rest design and an expanded pervasiveness of rest issues. Tending to the rest needs of these populaces is pivotal for advancing wellbeing across the life expectancy.

6.2 Discussing common sleep disorders and their solutions

Rest problems envelop a large number of conditions that upset the regular rest wake cycle, prompting challenges in nodding off, staying unconscious, or encountering helpful rest. These issues can essentially influence physical and emotional well-being, mental capability, and in general prosperity. In this extensive investigation, we will dig into normal rest issues, figuring out their basic causes, investigating their consequences for people, and talking about possible answers for relieve their effect.

One pervasive rest problem is sleep deprivation, portrayed by trouble nodding off, staying unconscious, or both. Sleep deprivation can be intense, going on for a brief period, or persistent, enduring over a lengthy span. It is frequently connected to different elements, including pressure, uneasiness, misery, and way of life decisions. The outcomes of sleep deprivation stretch out past simple weariness, influencing mental capability, state of mind, and by and large personal satisfaction.

The reasons for sleep deprivation are diverse, with mental, physiological, and natural variables assuming critical parts. Stress and nervousness, whether connected with work, connections, or other life altering situations, can add to a hyperactive brain that opposes unwinding. Also, unpredictable rest plans, unreasonable caffeine admission, and ecological factors, for example, commotion or light contamination can disturb the rest wake cycle, sustaining a sleeping disorder.

Mental Conduct Treatment for A sleeping disorder (CBT-I) has arisen as a profoundly powerful non-pharmacological methodology for overseeing a sleeping disorder. This helpful intercession centers around distinguishing and altering considerations and ways of behaving that add to rest troubles. CBT-I plans to further develop rest cleanliness, lay out a steady rest schedule, and address negative idea designs related with rest. By tending to the main drivers of a sleeping disorder, CBT-I offers feasible and long haul arrangements.

Another normal rest problem is rest apnea, a condition described by breaks in breathing during rest. There are two primary sorts of rest apnea: obstructive rest apnea (OSA) and focal rest apnea. OSA happens when the muscles in the throat unwind exorbitantly, prompting a fractional or complete blockage of the aviation route. Focal rest apnea, more uncommon, is described by the cerebrum's inability to convey appropriate messages to the muscles that control relaxing.

Untreated rest apnea can have serious wellbeing suggestions, including an expanded gamble of cardiovascular issues like hypertension, stroke, and coronary illness. The redundant patterns of oxygen hardship and excitement from rest can prompt daytime exhaustion, mental hindrance, and an in general decreased personal satisfaction. Constant Positive Aviation route Tension (CPAP) treatment is a typical treatment for rest apnea, including the utilization of a machine that conveys a ceaseless stream of air to keep the aviation route open.

Narcolepsy is a neurological problem that influences the cerebrum's capacity to manage rest wake cycles. People with narcolepsy might encounter abrupt and wild episodes of rest during the day, frequently joined by side effects, for example, cataplexy (unexpected loss of muscle tone), rest loss of motion, and distinctive fantasies. The specific reason for narcolepsy isn't completely perceived, however including a mix of hereditary and natural factors is thought.

Treatment for narcolepsy normally includes a blend of medicine and way of life changes. Energizer drugs, for example, modafinil or methylphenidate, can assist with advancing attentiveness and lighten exorbitant daytime drowsiness. Furthermore, energizer prescriptions might be endorsed to oversee side effects of cataplexy and further develop evening rest. Way of life changes, for example, keeping a predictable rest timetable and laying down for brief rests, can likewise add to better side effect the executives.

Fretful Legs Condition (RLS) is a neurological problem portrayed by a compelling desire to move the legs, frequently joined by awkward sensations like shivering or hurting. These side effects normally deteriorate during times of idleness, especially at night or around evening time, prompting challenges in nodding off. The specific reason for RLS isn't surely known, however both hereditary and natural elements are accepted to contribute.

The executives of RLS frequently includes way of life changes, for example, consolidating standard activity, embracing great rest cleanliness rehearses, and keeping away from substances that might worsen side effects, including caffeine and certain meds. In additional serious cases, prescriptions, for example, dopaminergic specialists, anticonvulsants, or narcotics might be endorsed to lighten side effects and further develop rest quality. Notwithstanding, the drawn out utilization of specific drugs requires cautious thought of likely aftereffects and dangers.

Shift Work Rest Problem (SWSD) is a circadian beat rest jumble that regularly influences people who work contemporary hours, for example, night moves or pivoting shifts. The disturbance of the normal circadian cadence, which is synchronized with the light-dim cycle, can prompt challenges in starting or keeping up with rest and a steady sensation of languor during work hours. SWSD is related with an expanded gamble of mishaps, impeded mental capability, and different medical problems.

Overseeing SWSD includes a mix of methodologies to further develop rest cleanliness and advance circadian cadence arrangement. Laying out a steady rest plan, establishing a dull and calm rest climate, and keeping away from energizers near sleep time can add to all the more likely rest quality. Light openness, especially openness to regular daylight, assumes a pivotal part in controlling the circadian musicality, and consolidating splendid light openness during work hours and limiting openness during the rest time frame can assist with moderating the impacts of SWSD.

Parasomnias incorporate a gathering of rest issues described by unusual ways of behaving, developments, or encounters during rest. Models incorporate sleepwalking, night fear, and REM rest conduct jumble (RBD). Parasomnias can be troublesome to the individual and, now and again, present dangers. They frequently happen during explicit rest arranges and might be affected by variables like hereditary qualities, meds, or other rest problems.

Treatment for parasomnias relies upon the particular issue and its seriousness. At times, tending to basic variables, like pressure or certain drugs, may lighten side effects. For sleepwalking, establishing a protected rest climate and carrying out unwinding methods might be valuable. In examples of RBD, where people showcase their fantasies during REM rest, drugs, for example, clonazepam might be recommended to lessen side effects and forestall wounds.

Investigating expected answers for rest problems includes a comprehensive methodology that thinks about both social and clinical mediations. Way of life changes, including embracing great rest cleanliness works on, keeping a predictable rest plan, and overseeing pressure, assume a vital part in further developing rest quality. Social treatments, like CBT-I, give successful apparatuses to tending to the hidden reasons for sleep deprivation and advancing feasible changes in rest designs.

Pharmacological mediations are frequently considered for specific rest problems, especially when non-pharmacological methodologies demonstrate lacking. Drugs might incorporate hypnotics for a sleeping disorder, energizers for narcolepsy, and prescriptions that address explicit side effects of parasomnias or development issues during rest. Be that as it may, the utilization of prescriptions ought to be drawn nearer warily, with cautious thought of expected incidental effects, reliance chances, and long haul suggestions.

Consistent Positive Aviation route Strain (CPAP) treatment stands apart as a profoundly compelling treatment for obstructive rest apnea. The CPAP machine conveys a persistent stream of air through a cover, forestalling aviation route breakdown and keeping up with typical breathing during rest. Adherence to CPAP treatment is essential for its viability, and people might go through a time of change as they become familiar with utilizing the gadget. Regardless of likely difficulties, CPAP treatment altogether further develops rest quality and decreases the related wellbeing dangers of untreated rest apnea.

Integrating normal actual work into day to day existence has been displayed to affect rest quality decidedly. Taking part in moderate-force work out, like strolling or cycling, can advance unwinding, decrease pressure, and add to more readily rest. Notwithstanding, it is vital for time actual work properly, staying away from overwhelming activity near sleep time, as it might make an invigorating difference and thwart the capacity to start rest.

Mind-body works on, including reflection, unwinding strategies, and yoga, offer successful devices for overseeing pressure and advancing unwinding. These practices can be integrated into a sleep time routine to flag the body that the time has come to slow down. Care reflection, specifically, has been related with upgrades in rest quality and can be a significant expansion to the collection of procedures for tending to rest issues.

Tending to rest problems requires a cooperative methodology including medical services experts, people, and, when pertinent, bosses. Looking for direction from medical care suppliers is vital for exact analysis and custom fitted therapy plans. Medical services experts might direct extensive rest appraisals, which can incorporate polysomnography (rest review) or home rest apnea testing, to assemble nitty gritty data about a singular's rest designs and recognize explicit rest issues.

6.3 Providing tips for improving sleep hygiene

Rest cleanliness alludes to a bunch of pursues and routines that advance sound rest and add to a serene night's rest. In our quick moving and frequently overwhelmed world, laying out great rest cleanliness is vital for generally speaking prosperity. This includes establishing a climate and taking on ways of behaving that help the body's normal rest wake cycle. In this nitty gritty investigation, we will dive into different methods for further developing rest cleanliness, enveloping both natural changes and way of life changes to cultivate a favorable climate for quality rest.

One key part of rest cleanliness is keeping a predictable rest plan. Hitting the sack and awakening simultaneously consistently, even on ends of the week, directs the body's inner clock. This consistency supports the normal circadian cadence, adjusting the rest wake cycle with the day-night cycle. Sporadic rest designs, like regularly switching sleep time or wake-around times, can upset this mood, prompting challenges nodding off or staying unconscious.

Making a loosening up sleep time routine is one more key part of compelling rest cleanliness. Taking part in quieting exercises before sleep time signs to the body that now is the ideal time to slow down. This could incorporate exercises, for example, perusing a book, washing up, rehearsing unwinding activities, or paying attention to mitigating music. Laying out a normal aides train the body to perceive prompts that go before rest, making it more straightforward to progress into a serene state.

The rest climate assumes a huge part in rest cleanliness. The room ought to be an agreeable and welcoming space devoted to rest and unwinding. Keeping a cool, dim, and calm climate can improve rest quality. Consider utilizing power outage draperies to shut out outer light, and use earplugs or a repetitive sound to limit unsettling influences from encompassing commotion. Putting resources into an agreeable bedding and cushions that offer legitimate help adds to a more peaceful rest insight.

Restricting openness to screens before sleep time is a vital part of present day rest cleanliness. The blue light radiated by cell phones, tablets, PCs, and TVs can smother the creation of melatonin, the rest instigating chemical. In a perfect world, keeping away from screens basically an hour prior to bedtime is suggested. On the off chance that this isn't achievable, utilizing blue light channels or "night mode" settings on gadgets can assist with alleviating the effect on melatonin creation.

The effect of caffeine on rest is deeply grounded, and directing its utilization is fundamental for good rest cleanliness. Caffeine is an energizer tracked down in espresso, tea, chocolate, and certain meds.

It can disrupt the capacity to nod off and decrease rest quality. Restricting caffeine consumption, particularly in the early evening and evening is fitting. Deciding on decaffeinated refreshments during the last option some portion of the day can be a shrewd decision for those delicate to caffeine's belongings.

Liquor, notwithstanding its underlying narcotic impacts, can upset the rest cycle and debilitate in general rest quality. While it might assist people with nodding off more rapidly, liquor slows down the later phases of rest, prompting more divided and less helpful rest. Directing liquor consumption, particularly in the hours paving the way to sleep time, adds to more readily rest cleanliness.

Normal active work has been connected to further developed rest quality, and integrating exercise into a day to day schedule is gainful for rest cleanliness. Taking part in moderate-force work out, like lively strolling or cycling, can advance unwinding and decrease pressure. In any case, it's vital to time actual work suitably, as energetic activity near sleep time might make an animating difference and obstruct the capacity to start rest.

Overseeing pressure and tension is fundamental for compelling rest cleanliness. Elevated degrees of stress enact the body's "instinctive" reaction, delivering pressure chemicals that can obstruct the capacity to unwind and nod off. Embracing pressure lessening procedures, like care reflection, profound breathing activities, or yoga, can assist with making a more quiet mental state helpful for rest.

Assessing and changing the rest climate is a down to earth move toward further developing rest cleanliness. The room ought to be helpful for rest, with an agreeable sleeping pad and cushions. Guaranteeing the room is cool, dim, and calm adds to an environment that welcomes rests. Moreover, limiting mess and making an outwardly quieting space can improve the general rest climate.

Restricting rests, or decisively integrating them into the everyday daily practice, is significant for keeping up with great rest cleanliness. While short rests can give a speedy jolt of energy, longer or unpredictably coordinated rests can impede the capacity to nod off around evening time. On the off chance that rests are business as usual, it's prudent to keep them brief (20-30 minutes) and timetable them prior in the day to try not to disturb the evening rest plan.

Staying away from enormous dinners near sleep time upholds great rest cleanliness. Processing a weighty feast can be awkward and may cause heartburn or reflux, making it trying to sufficiently rest. It's prescribed to have a light tidbit if hungry before sleep time, picking food varieties that advance unwinding, like a little serving of nuts, yogurt, or a banana.

Keeping an agreeable room temperature is essential for a soothing rest climate. The ideal temperature might shift from one individual to another, yet it for the most part falls somewhere in the range of 60 and 67 degrees Fahrenheit (15-20 degrees Celsius). Exploring different avenues regarding bedding and attire layers permits people to find the ideal mix that guarantees they stay serenely cool over the course of the evening.

For people battling with sleep deprivation or trouble nodding off, it's significant not to invest an excessive amount of energy in bed conscious. In the event that unfit to nod off inside around 20-30 minutes, it's fitting to get up and participate in a peaceful, loosening up movement until feeling tired. This helps break the relationship between the bed and attentiveness, advancing a more powerful rest wake cycle.

Mental Social Treatment for A sleeping disorder (CBT-I) is an organized and proof based helpful methodology for tending to rest challenges. CBT-I targets considerations and ways of behaving that add to a sleeping disorder, planning to supplant them with better examples. Methods might incorporate improvement control (connecting the bed with rest), rest limitation (restricting time spent in bed alert), and mental rebuilding (changing negative contemplations about rest).

In situations where rest troubles persevere notwithstanding executing great rest cleanliness rehearses, it is essential to look for proficient assistance. Medical services suppliers, including essential consideration doctors and rest subject matter experts, can direct far reaching rest appraisals to distinguish hidden issues. Polysomnography (rest studies) might be prescribed to assemble nitty gritty data about rest designs and analyze explicit rest issues.

Melatonin supplements, a normally happening chemical that directs the rest wake cycle, can be considered for specific rest issues. Melatonin supplements are available without a prescription and may assist people with circadian mood unsettling influences or hardships changing in accordance with changes in rest plans, like fly slack. It's vital to utilize melatonin supplements under the direction of a medical care proficient, as measurements and timing are basic for viability.

For people determined to have rest problems, for example, rest apnea, ceaseless positive aviation route pressure (CPAP) treatment is a profoundly powerful treatment. CPAP includes the utilization of a machine that conveys a consistent stream of air through a cover, forestalling aviation route breakdown during rest. Adherence to CPAP treatment is significant for its prosperity, and people might go through a change period as they become acquainted with utilizing the gadget.

Way of life changes and conduct mediations assume a urgent part in overseeing rest issues. Weight reduction, for instance, can be helpful for people with rest apnea, as abundance weight can add to aviation route block during rest.

Stopping smoking is one more significant stage, as smoking has been connected to rest unsettling influences and an expanded gamble of rest problems.

Integrating unwinding strategies into the sleep time routine is useful for people with sleep deprivation or uplifted feelings of anxiety. Care reflection, moderate muscle unwinding, or directed symbolism can assist with quieting the brain and decrease tension, making a more helpful climate for nodding off. These procedures are important for the more extensive system of further developing rest cleanliness by encouraging unwinding before sleep time.

The significance of rest cleanliness stretches out to explicit populaces, including youngsters and more established grown-ups. Laying out great rest propensities since the beginning is critical for youngsters' turn of events and prosperity. Steady sleep time schedules, restricting screen time, and establishing a rest favorable climate add to solid rest cleanliness for youngsters. More seasoned grown-ups may confront one of a kind difficulties connected with rest, for example, changes in rest engineering and an expanded predominance of specific rest problems. Changing rest schedules, consolidating active work, and tending to fundamental medical problems are fundamental for advancing rest cleanliness in this segment.

All in all, focusing on great rest cleanliness is a central stage toward guaranteeing peaceful and supportive rest. The transaction of ecological changes and way of life changes makes an extensive way to deal with cultivating a climate that welcomes rests. From keeping a steady rest timetable to overseeing pressure, embracing these tips can essentially add to further developed rest quality and in general prosperity. As people, families, and networks embrace the significance of rest cleanliness.

Upgrading rest cleanliness is a complex undertaking that includes taking on a bunch of pursues and routines to improve the quality and term of rest. In a world set apart by consistent network and requesting plans, focusing on rest cleanliness turns out to be progressively critical for generally prosperity. This complete investigation dives into different methodologies and way of life changes that add to further developed rest cleanliness, incorporating both ecological and social contemplations.

Prescription For A Healthy Life

Consistency in rest designs is a foundation of powerful rest cleanliness. Laying out a standard rest plan includes heading to sleep and awakening simultaneously consistently, even on ends of the week. This consistency manages the body's interior clock, adjusting the rest wake cycle with the normal circadian musicality. Unpredictable rest designs, like habitually switching sleep time or wake-around times, can disturb this arrangement, prompting troubles nodding off or staying unconscious.

Making a quieting sleep time routine is an important part of rest cleanliness. Taking part in loosening up exercises before sleep time signs to the body that now is the ideal time to slow down.

This routine could incorporate perusing a book, washing up, rehearsing care reflection, or paying attention to relieving music. Laying out a reliable sleep time routine trains the body to perceive prompts that go before rest, working with a smoother change into a relaxing state.

The rest climate assumes an essential part in rest cleanliness. The room ought to be an agreeable and welcoming space committed to rest and unwinding. Keeping a cool, dull, and calm climate improves rest quality. Consider utilizing power outage draperies to shut out outside light, and use earplugs or a repetitive sound to limit unsettling influences from surrounding commotion. Putting resources into an agreeable bedding and pads that offer satisfactory help adds to a more soothing rest insight.

Lessening screen time before sleep time is a urgent part of current rest cleanliness. The blue light discharged by cell phones, tablets, PCs, and TVs can smother the creation of melatonin, a chemical that controls rest. In a perfect world, keeping away from screens basically an hour prior to bedtime is suggested. In the event that this isn't possible, utilizing blue light channels or "night mode" settings on gadgets can assist with alleviating the effect on melatonin creation.

The effect of caffeine on rest is proven and factual, and directing its utilization is fundamental for good rest cleanliness. Caffeine, an energizer tracked down in espresso, tea, chocolate, and certain prescriptions, can obstruct the capacity to nod off and decrease rest quality. Restricting caffeine admission, particularly in the early evening and night, adds to further developed rest cleanliness. Picking decaffeinated drinks during the last option some portion of the day is an insightful decision for those delicate to caffeine's belongings.

Liquor, notwithstanding its underlying narcotic impacts, can upset the rest cycle and weaken generally rest quality. While it might assist people with nodding off more rapidly, liquor disrupts the later phases of rest, prompting more divided and less helpful rest. Directing liquor admission, particularly in the hours paving the way to sleep time, adds to more readily rest cleanliness.

Customary active work is connected to further developed rest quality and is an essential part of rest cleanliness. Taking part in moderate-power work out, like energetic strolling or cycling, advances unwinding and lessens pressure. Be that as it may, it's fundamental for time actual work suitably, as fiery activity near sleep time might make an invigorating difference and obstruct the capacity to start rest.

Stress the executives is a urgent component of viable rest cleanliness. Elevated degrees of stress actuate the body's "survival" reaction, delivering pressure chemicals that can slow down the capacity to unwind and nod off. Embracing pressure diminishing procedures, like care reflection, profound breathing activities, or yoga, can assist with making a more peaceful mental state helpful for rest.

The rest climate is a pragmatic point of convergence for further developing rest cleanliness. Assessing and changing components inside the room add to making an ideal setting for rest. The sleeping pad and cushions ought to be agreeable and steady, and the room temperature ought to be cool and agreeable. Guaranteeing the room is dull and calm, and limiting mess, upgrades the general rest climate.

Restricting daytime snoozing or decisively consolidating short rests is a fundamental thought for keeping up with great rest cleanliness. While short rests can give a fast jolt of energy, longer or unpredictably planned rests can impede the capacity to nod off around evening time. Assuming that rests are business as usual, keeping them brief (20-30 minutes) and booking them prior in the day evades disturbance to the evening rest plan.

Staying away from huge feasts near sleep time is a down to earth methodology for supporting great rest cleanliness. Processing a weighty feast can be awkward and may cause heartburn or reflux, making it trying to sufficiently rest. Deciding on a light bite if hungry before sleep time is fitting, picking food sources that advance unwinding, like a little serving of nuts, yogurt, or a banana.

Keeping an agreeable room temperature is indispensable for establishing a relaxing rest climate. The ideal temperature might fluctuate from one individual to another, yet it for the most part falls somewhere in the range of 60 and 67 degrees Fahrenheit (15-20 degrees Celsius). Exploring different avenues regarding bedding and attire layers permits people to find the ideal blend that guarantees they stay serenely cool over the course of the evening.

For people encountering trouble nodding off, it's urgent not to invest an excessive amount of energy in bed alert. If unfit to nod off inside around 20-30 minutes, getting up and participating in a peaceful, loosening up movement until feeling languid is fitting. This approach helps break the relationship between the bed and attentiveness, advancing a more compelling rest wake cycle.

Mental Conduct Treatment for Sleep deprivation (CBT-I) is an organized and proof based restorative methodology for tending to rest challenges. CBT-I targets considerations and ways of behaving that add to sleep deprivation, expecting to supplant them with better examples. Procedures might incorporate boost control (connecting the bed with rest), rest limitation (restricting time spent in bed conscious), and mental rebuilding (changing negative contemplations about rest).

Prescription For A Healthy Life

In situations where rest troubles persevere in spite of executing great rest cleanliness rehearses, it is vital to look for proficient assistance. Medical services suppliers, including essential consideration doctors and rest trained professionals, can lead exhaustive rest evaluations to distinguish basic issues. Polysomnography (rest studies) might be prescribed to assemble point by point data about rest designs and analyze explicit rest problems.

Melatonin supplements, a normally happening chemical that controls the rest wake cycle, can be considered for specific rest issues. Melatonin supplements are available without a prescription and may assist people with circadian cadence aggravations or hardships acclimating to changes in rest plans, like fly slack. It's essential to utilize melatonin supplements under the direction of a medical care proficient, as measurements and timing are basic for viability.

For people determined to have rest problems, for example, rest apnea, ceaseless positive aviation route pressure (CPAP) treatment is an exceptionally viable treatment. CPAP includes the utilization of a machine that conveys a persistent stream of air through a veil, forestalling aviation route breakdown during rest. Adherence to CPAP treatment is significant for its prosperity, and people might go through a change period as they become acquainted with utilizing the gadget.

Way of life changes and conduct mediations assume a urgent part in overseeing rest issues. Weight reduction, for instance, can be helpful for people with rest apnea, as overabundance weight can add to aviation route obstacle during rest. Stopping smoking is one more significant stage, as smoking has been connected to rest aggravations and an expanded gamble of rest problems.

Integrating unwinding procedures into the sleep time routine is advantageous for people with sleep deprivation or uplifted feelings of anxiety. Care contemplation, moderate muscle unwinding, or directed symbolism can assist with quieting the psyche and lessen uneasiness, making a more helpful climate for nodding off. These procedures are essential for the more extensive system of further developing rest cleanliness by cultivating unwinding before sleep time.

The significance of rest cleanliness reaches out to explicit populaces, including youngsters and more seasoned grown-ups. Laying out great rest propensities since the beginning is urgent for youngsters' turn of events and prosperity. Reliable sleep time schedules, restricting screen time, and establishing a rest favorable climate add to solid rest cleanliness for kids. More established grown-ups may confront one of a kind difficulties connected with rest, for example, changes in rest engineering and an expanded predominance of specific rest issues. Changing rest schedules, consolidating active work, and tending to fundamental medical problems are fundamental for advancing rest cleanliness in this segment.

Chapter 7

Building Healthy Habits

Building sound propensities is a long lasting excursion that requires commitment, care, and a readiness to roll out certain improvements in different parts of our lives. Whether it's working on actual wellbeing, developing a positive outlook, or encouraging significant associations, the underpinning of a sound way of life lies in the propensities we develop consistently.

One of the principal mainstays of building solid propensities is ordinary actual work. Practice adds to actual prosperity as well as assumes a pivotal part in keeping up with emotional wellness. Taking part in various exercises, from cardiovascular activities like running or cycling to strength preparing and adaptability works out, assists with keeping the body spry and strong. The key is to track down exercises that one appreciates, making it simpler to integrate them into a day to day daily schedule.

Notwithstanding organized work out, taking on a functioning way of life can significantly affect by and large wellbeing. Straightforward decisions like using the stairwell rather than the lift, strolling or cycling as opposed to driving for brief distances, and integrating development into day to day undertakings add to expanded actual work levels. These little changes, when reliably applied, amount to make a better, more dynamic way of life.

Sustenance is one more basic part of building sound propensities. An even eating routine that incorporates different supplement thick food sources is fundamental for ideal physical and mental working. Underlining organic products, vegetables, entire grains, lean proteins, and solid fats furnishes the body with the fundamental supplements to flourish. Segment control is likewise crucial to forestall gorging and keep a solid weight.

Hydration is frequently disregarded yet is a central part of a sound way of life. Drinking a satisfactory measure of water over the course of the day upholds different physical processes, including assimilation, supplement retention, and temperature guideline. Fostering the propensity for conveying a reusable water container and putting forth a cognizant attempt to remain hydrated is a basic yet viable move toward generally speaking prosperity.

Sufficient rest is a foundation of good wellbeing. Laying out a reliable rest routine and guaranteeing that one gets the suggested measure of rest every night is pivotal for physical and mental recuperation. Quality rest adds to further developed temperament, mental capability, and in general flexibility to push. Establishing a helpful rest climate, rehearsing unwinding procedures, and restricting screen time before sleep time are techniques that can advance better rest.

Care and stress the board are indispensable parts of building solid propensities. Persistent pressure can inconveniently affect both physical and emotional wellness. Integrating practices like contemplation, profound breathing activities, or yoga into everyday schedules oversees feelings of anxiety and advances a feeling of quiet and equilibrium. Developing care includes being available at the time, appreciating the little delights of life, and creating flexibility notwithstanding challenges.

Fabricating and keeping up with positive connections is a critical component of a sound way of life. Social associations offer profound help, diminish sensations of dejection, and add to in general prosperity. Investing energy with friends and family, developing kinships, and participating in significant discussions add to a feeling of having a place and satisfaction. Sustaining solid connections includes viable correspondence, compassion, and the ability to put time and exertion in building associations.

Defining and pursuing significant objectives is a strong inspiration for building solid propensities. Whether it's wellness objectives, profession yearnings, or self-improvement goals, having an unmistakable feeling of direction gives guidance and inspiration.

Separating bigger objectives into more modest, reachable advances gains ground more reasonable and manageable. Commending accomplishments en route supports positive propensities and lifts certainty.

Using time effectively is a basic calculate the excursion to a better way of life. Adjusting work, individual life, and taking care of oneself requires deliberate preparation and prioritization. Making a timetable that considers committed time for work out, feast readiness, unwinding, and rest guarantees that wellbeing related exercises are focused on. Powerful using time effectively likewise includes perceiving when to designate undertakings, express no to extra responsibilities, and focus on taking care of oneself.

Consistency is the way to building and keeping up with solid propensities. Laying out a standard that consolidates different parts of physical and mental prosperity guarantees that sound ways of behaving become imbued in day to day existence. Predictable exertion over the long haul prompts enduring positive changes. It's critical to move toward the cycle with persistence and versatility, perceiving that difficulties are a characteristic piece of the excursion.

Adjusting to change is a fundamental expertise chasing a solid way of life. Life is dynamic, and conditions might advance, expecting acclimations to schedules and propensities. Adaptability and a readiness to adjust to new circumstances add to long haul progress in building and keeping up with solid propensities. As opposed to review change as a hindrance, developing an outlook that embraces valuable open doors for development and transformation is urgent.

Mindfulness is a foundation of building sound propensities. Figuring out one's qualities, assets, and regions for development gives understanding into the inspirations driving way of life decisions. Customary self-reflection permits people to survey their headway, distinguish areas of development, and make changes depending on the situation. Developing mindfulness includes focusing on physical and close to home prompts, perceiving examples of conduct, and pursuing cognizant decisions lined up with individual qualities.

Building solid propensities stretches out past individual prosperity to incorporate natural manageability. Going with eco-cognizant decisions, like diminishing single-utilize plastic, saving energy, and supporting reasonable practices, adds to the general wellbeing of the planet. Perceiving the interconnectedness of individual wellbeing and the strength of the climate elevates an all encompassing way to deal with prosperity.

Training and nonstop learning assume a crucial part in building and keeping up with sound propensities. Remaining informed about the most recent examination, health patterns, and proof based rehearses engages people to go with informed decisions. Searching out dependable wellsprings of data, talking with medical services experts, and staying open to novel thoughts add to a balanced way to deal with wellbeing and prosperity.

Building solid propensities is a deep rooted responsibility that requires continuous exertion and versatility. The excursion is interesting to every person, impacted by private qualities, needs, and conditions. Embracing the cycle as a ceaseless development, instead of an objective, cultivates a mentality that empowers development and strength. By focusing on active work, sustenance, rest, care, and positive connections, people can make an establishment for a sound and satisfying life.

All in all, the excursion to building solid propensities envelops different elements of prosperity, including actual wellbeing, mental flexibility, and positive connections. Normal active work, a decent eating routine, hydration, and adequate rest structure the premise of actual prosperity. Care, stress the board, and positive social associations add to mental and profound wellbeing. Defining significant objectives, overseeing time actually, and embracing change are fundamental for supported progress. Consistency, mindfulness, and a promise to long lasting learning are pivotal components of an all encompassing way to deal with building and keeping up with sound propensities. At last, the quest for a sound way of life is a dynamic and continuous cycle that requires devotion, self-reflection, and an eagerness to adjust to the consistently changing nature of life.

7.1 Discussing the science of habit formation

Diving into the study of propensity development uncovers an intriguing transaction of mental, neurological, and social factors that shape our schedules and ways of behaving. Understanding the fundamental instruments of propensity arrangement is urgent for anybody looking to develop positive propensities or break liberated from unfavorable ones.

Propensities are basically programmed ways of behaving that are procured through redundancy. The course of propensity development includes a circle of signal, everyday practice, and prize. The prompt goes about as a trigger, flagging the mind to start a particular way of behaving or schedule. This routine is the ongoing conduct itself, and it is trailed by a prize, which supports the association between the signal and the daily practice. Over the long haul, as this circle is rehashed, the propensity becomes imbued in the brain connections of the cerebrum.

The mind assumes a focal part in propensity development, with a central member being the basal ganglia, a locale related with coordinated movements and procedural learning. As propensities become more instilled, the basal ganglia assumes control over the execution of the way of behaving, opening up the prefrontal cortex, the region liable for navigation and cognizant idea, to zero in on additional complicated errands. This change in brain handling makes propensities programmed and less dependent on cognizant exertion.

Synapses, like dopamine, likewise assume a pivotal part in propensity development. Dopamine is a synapse related with joy and prize, and its delivery builds up the association between the everyday practice and the good inclination related with finishing the way of behaving. This support adds to the foundation and upkeep of propensities.

The idea of brain adaptability further accentuates the cerebrum's capacity to adjust and change after some time. As propensities are shaped, brain associations are fortified, and the cerebrum goes through primary changes to oblige the dull way of behaving. Understanding the brain adaptability of the cerebrum gives experiences into the flexibility of propensities and the potential for reworking brain connections to lay out better schedules.

Natural prompts, or triggers, likewise assume a huge part in propensity development. These prompts can be outer, like a particular area or season of day, or inside, similar to a profound state. The consistency of these prompts hardens the propensity circle by making an anticipated example that the mind perceives and answers. Distinguishing and controlling these prompts can be a strong technique for both laying out new propensities and breaking liberated from unwanted ones.

The job of criticism in propensity development couldn't possibly be more significant. Quick and positive criticism upgrades the probability of propensity development, as the mind connects the way of behaving with a pleasurable result. In actuality, postponed or negative criticism can ruin the cycle, as the cerebrum might battle to lay out an unmistakable association between the way of behaving and its ramifications.

To effectively develop positive propensities, zeroing in on establishing a favorable climate that upholds the ideal behavior is fundamental. Eliminating snags and making the ideal way of behaving as helpful as potential improves the probability of propensity arrangement. This lines up with the idea of "ecological plan" or "decision design," where the physical and social climate is purposefully molded to support explicit ways of behaving.

The length expected to lay out a propensity shifts generally among people and ways of behaving. The well known idea that it requires 21 days to shape a propensity has been tested by research proposing that the time span is more nuanced and setting subordinate. The intricacy of propensity development, affected by elements like the trouble of the way of behaving and individual contrasts, highlights the significance of tolerance and perseverance simultaneously.

Ending liberated from unwanted propensities includes a comparable comprehension of the propensity circle yet requires deliberate interruption. Distinguishing the sign that sets off the undesirable way of behaving is a pivotal initial step. When the prompt is perceived, deliberately modifying the standard that observes can assist with disturbing the propensity circle. This interaction, known as "propensity inversion," includes subbing the unfortunate way of behaving with a more sure one, preferably one that actually gives a feeling of remuneration.

The study of propensity arrangement has additionally been applied in helpful settings, especially in medicines like Mental Conduct Treatment (CBT). CBT underlines recognizing and adjusting examples of conduct, including propensities, to advance positive psychological well-being results.

By figuring out the signals, schedules, and rewards related with maladaptive ways of behaving, people can work with specialists to foster methodologies for bringing an end to liberated from pessimistic propensities and laying out better other options.

The idea of cornerstone propensities adds one more layer to the comprehension of propensity development. Cornerstone propensities are explicit ways of behaving that, when taken on, have an expanding influence, decidedly impacting different everyday issues. For instance, ordinary activity is many times considered a cornerstone propensity since it will in general prompt superior rest, better dietary patterns, and expanded by and large prosperity. Zeroing in on developing cornerstone propensities can give an essential way to deal with starting positive change.

Prescription For A Healthy Life

Social impact and the force of informal organizations likewise assume a critical part in propensity development. Ways of behaving can be infectious, and people are bound to embrace propensities assuming they see others in their groups of friends doing as such. Utilizing the positive impact of social associations can upgrade the probability of fruitful propensity development. Alternately, understanding the effect of negative social impacts is critical for staying away from the reception of unfortunate things to do.

The connection among propensities and self discipline is a complex and frequently misjudged part of conduct change. While determination can be a significant asset for starting change, depending entirely on resolution to keep up with propensities is in many cases impractical in the long haul. Propensities, when shaped, become programmed and less reliant upon cognizant exertion. In this way, building propensities decisively, considering the study of propensity arrangement, can assist with moderating self discipline for additional difficult undertakings.

The effect of propensities reaches out past individual prosperity to cultural and social levels. Social standards and cultural assumptions impact the propensities people take on, forming the general wellbeing and prosperity of networks. General wellbeing drives frequently center around advancing positive propensities at a cultural level, perceiving the aggregate effect of propensities on the strength of populaces.

Innovation plays likewise had an impact in forming propensities, both decidedly and adversely. The universality of cell phones and applications has given new instruments to propensity development, offering updates, following advancement, and giving input. Nonetheless, the habit-forming nature of innovation, especially web-based entertainment and online stages, has additionally led to propensities that might have adverse results on emotional well-being and efficiency.

All in all, the study of propensity development offers an exhaustive comprehension of the mental, neurological, and social factors that impact our schedules and ways of behaving.

Propensities, whether positive or negative, are profoundly imbued in the brain processes of the mind, formed by signs, schedules, and rewards. The interchange of natural prompts, brain adaptability, input, and social impacts adds to the intricacy of propensity arrangement.

Applying this logical information to the development of positive propensities includes deliberate natural plan, recognizing and controlling signs, and utilizing the force of criticism. Bringing an end to liberated from unfortunate propensities requires a comparable comprehension of the propensity circle, alongside purposeful disturbance and propensity inversion methodologies. The span expected to lay out a propensity changes among people and ways of behaving, stressing the requirement for tolerance and perseverance simultaneously.

Cornerstone propensities, social impact, and the connection among propensities and resolve add profundity to the investigation of propensity development. Perceiving the cultural and social effect of propensities highlights the significance of thinking about propensities at a more extensive level, past individual way of behaving. As innovation keeps on deeply shaping our day to day routines, understanding its job in propensity development turns out to be progressively significant.

Eventually, the study of propensity arrangement gives significant bits of knowledge to anybody trying to start positive conduct change. Whether in self-improvement, helpful settings, or general wellbeing drives, applying this information decisively can upgrade the probability of outcome in building and keeping up with sound propensities.

7.2 Providing practical advice on building and sustaining healthy habits

Setting out on the excursion of building and supporting sound propensities requires an insightful and comprehensive methodology. While the study of propensity development gives significant experiences, viable counsel custom-made to individual requirements and inclinations is fundamental for long haul achievement. This direction envelops different parts of prosperity, including actual wellbeing, mental flexibility, and positive way of life decisions.

A fundamental component in building solid propensities is standard active work. Notwithstanding, the key is to track down exercises that one appreciates and that line up with individual inclinations and wellness levels. Whether it's running, swimming, moving, or rehearsing yoga, the objective is to make practice a charming and feasible piece of day to day existence. Begin progressively, integrating exercises into the everyday practice and step by step expanding power to stay balanced or injury.

Consistency is foremost in the domain of active work. Laying out a standard that incorporates assigned times for practice helps make it a non-debatable piece of day to day existence.

Consistency cements the propensity as well as adds to the combined advantages of normal activity. Whether it's a morning run, a noon exercise, or a night yoga meeting, figure out an opportunity that works best and focus on it reliably.

Defining practical and feasible objectives is an essential part of building sound propensities, including those connected with actual work. Separate bigger wellness objectives into more modest, reasonable advances. Celebrate accomplishments en route, whether it's finishing a specific distance, arriving at a particular weight-lifting objective, or dominating another yoga present. Perceiving progress builds up certain propensities and keeps inspiration high.

Nourishment is one more foundation of a solid way of life. Embracing a decent and shifted diet that incorporates a range of supplements is fundamental for generally speaking prosperity. Center around integrating entire food sources like organic products, vegetables, lean proteins, entire grains, and solid fats into feasts.

Explore different avenues regarding various recipes and cooking strategies to keep the eating regimen intriguing and maintainable.

Dinner arranging and arrangement can essentially add to building and supporting smart dieting propensities. Put away opportunity every week to design dinners, make a shopping list, and get ready nutritious fixings. Having sound choices promptly accessible decreases the compulsion to decide on less nutritious other options. Consider bunch cooking to save time during occupied days and guarantee admittance to supporting feasts.

Hydration is frequently neglected yet is an essential part of keeping up with great wellbeing. Drinking a sufficient measure of water upholds different physical processes, including assimilation, supplement ingestion, and temperature guideline. Practice it regularly to convey a reusable water jug and set suggestions to hydrate over the course of the day. Seasoning water with a sprinkle of lemon or implanting it with natural products can make hydration more pleasant.

Satisfactory rest is a mainstay of prosperity that ought to be considered carefully. Laying out a reliable rest schedule, including a standard sleep time and wake-up time, adds to more readily rest quality. Establish a rest favorable climate by keeping the room dull, calm, and cool. Limit screen time before bed and practice unwinding strategies, like profound breathing or reflection, to advance soothing rest.

Care and stress the executives are necessary parts of building and supporting sound propensities. Integrate practices like reflection, profound breathing activities, or yoga into everyday schedules to oversee feelings of anxiety actually. Care includes being available at the time, appreciating the little delights of life, and creating flexibility despite challenges. Find care procedures that reverberate and coordinate them into day to day existence.

Developing positive connections is a vital part of a sound way of life. Encircling oneself with steady and elevating people cultivates profound prosperity and gives a feeling of association. Put time and exertion in supporting significant associations with family, companions, and partners. Participate in exercises that reinforce social bonds, whether it's a common leisure activity, a normal get together, or a genuine discussion.

Compelling correspondence is essential in building and supporting positive connections. Offering viewpoints, sentiments, and needs straightforwardly and sincerely adds to understanding and association. Effectively pay attention to other people, practice sympathy, and be open to criticism. Sound connections include coordinated effort, split the difference, and shared regard, establishing a climate that upholds by and large prosperity.

Defining limits is a significant part of keeping up with sound connections and individual prosperity. Obviously characterize limits in regards to time, energy, and responsibilities. Figuring out how to say no when vital and focusing on taking care of oneself forestalls burnout and guarantees that individual wellbeing stays a need. Conscious openness is absolutely vital while laying out and discussing limits with others.

Objective setting reaches out past actual wellbeing to include different parts of individual and expert turn of events. Setting explicit, quantifiable, feasible, significant, and time-bound (Brilliant) objectives gives an unmistakable guide to advance. Whether it's progressing in a profession, chasing after instructive open doors, or dominating another expertise, clear cut objectives make heading and inspiration.

Compelling using time productively is essential chasing a sound way of life. Focus on undertakings in light of significance and criticalness, dispense time for different exercises, and make a timetable that considers balance between work, individual life, and taking care of oneself. Perceive when to assign undertakings, look for help, and when to enjoy reprieves to forestall burnout. Reliably rehearsing great using time effectively adds to in general prosperity.

Reliable self-reflection is an amazing asset in building and supporting sound propensities. Consistently survey individual qualities, needs, and objectives to guarantee arrangement with day to day decisions and ways of behaving. Perceive examples of conduct, both positive and negative, and make cognizant changes on a case by case basis. Developing mindfulness gives knowledge into inspirations and cultivates self-improvement.

Adjusting to change is an inborn piece of life, and adaptability is an important expertise in building and supporting solid propensities. Embrace change as a chance for development, perceiving that conditions might advance, expecting acclimations to schedules and propensities. An outlook that embraces flexibility and perspectives change as a characteristic piece of the excursion adds to long haul achievement.

Persistent learning is an essential part of self-improvement and propensity arrangement. Remain informed about the most recent exploration, health patterns, and proof based rehearses. Search out dependable wellsprings of data, talk with medical care experts, and stay open to groundbreaking thoughts and approaches. A readiness to learn and adjust adds to a balanced and informed way to deal with wellbeing and prosperity.

Fabricating and supporting sound propensities additionally include natural contemplations. Pursue decisions that line up with manageability and backing the prosperity of the planet. Decrease single-utilize plastic, ration energy, and backing eco-accommodating practices. Perceiving the interconnectedness of individual wellbeing and natural wellbeing elevates a comprehensive way to deal with prosperity.

The excursion to building and supporting sound propensities is a dynamic and progressing process that requires commitment, self-reflection, and an eagerness to adjust. It includes deliberate decisions in different parts of life, from actual work and nourishment to rest, care, and connections. By integrating viable guidance customized to individual requirements, people can make an establishment for a solid and satisfying life.

All in all, building and supporting sound propensities envelop a multi-layered approach that tends to actual wellbeing, mental versatility, positive connections, and way of life decisions. Down to earth guidance incorporates tracking down pleasant types of active work, putting forth reasonable objectives, embracing a fair and changed diet, focusing on hydration and rest, rehearsing care, developing positive connections, viable correspondence, defining limits, objective setting, using time productively, self-reflection, versatility, nonstop learning, and natural contemplations. By integrating these components into day to day existence, people can leave on an excursion that forms solid propensities as well as cultivates a supportable and satisfying way of life.

7.3 Addressing common obstacles and how to overcome them

Leaving on the excursion to construct and support solid propensities is without a doubt fulfilling, however it isn't without its difficulties. Normal snags can block progress and wreck endeavors to make positive way of life changes. Figuring out these moves and carrying out compelling techniques to conquer them is fundamental for long haul progress in developing a sound and satisfying life.

One predominant snag is the absence of inspiration. Inspiration will in general change, and people might find it trying to support excitement for their wellbeing objectives over the long run. To address this, distinguishing individual inspirations that go past shallow desires is urgent. Interfacing wellbeing objectives to more profound qualities, for example, needing to be available for friends and family or working on generally speaking prosperity, can give a really persevering through wellspring of inspiration.

Also, setting explicit, quantifiable, and reachable objectives can upgrade inspiration. Separating bigger objectives into more modest, reasonable advances considers a feeling of achievement en route. Praising these little triumphs supports positive propensities and adds to a positive input circle, helping generally speaking inspiration.

Another normal impediment is an absence of time, frequently refered to as an obstruction to participating in sound ways of behaving like activity, dinner planning, and taking care of oneself. To defeat time imperatives, it's fundamental to intentionally focus on and plan exercises. Time usage methodologies, for example, making an everyday or week by week plan, can assist with dispensing time for work out, dinner arranging, and other wellbeing related exercises.

Integrating actual work into everyday schedules, like using the stairwell rather than the lift or taking a stroll during breaks, is a reasonable method for beating time limits. Moreover, consolidating exercises, like associating while at the same time practicing or getting ready dinners in clusters to save time, can be compelling in boosting accessible time.

Another critical impediment is the appeal of moment satisfaction over long haul benefits. Unfortunate propensities frequently give prompt joy or help, making it trying to decide on better options that may not yield moment results. Beating this deterrent includes moving the concentration from momentary prizes to long haul prosperity.

Developing care is a strong methodology to address the charm of moment satisfaction. Care includes being available at the time and going with cognizant decisions. By stopping and taking into account the drawn out results of decisions, people can pursue choices that line up with their wellbeing objectives. Careful eating, for instance, includes enjoying each chomp and focusing on craving and completion signs, advancing better dietary patterns.

Stalling is one more typical obstacle on the way to building sound propensities. Postponing the inception of new propensities or putting off practice meetings can frustrate progress. Defeating tarrying requires understanding its main drivers, which might incorporate feeling of dread toward disappointment, absence of certainty, or a feeling of overpower.

Separating errands into more modest, more reasonable advances can help ease the overpower related with taking on new propensities. Making a definite arrangement, setting cutoff times, and utilizing instruments like plans for the day or propensity following applications can give construction and responsibility. Furthermore, looking for help from companions, family, or a wellbeing expert can offer support and help with beating tarrying.

Conflicting or unreasonable objective setting is another impediment that can block progress. Putting forth excessively aggressive objectives or continually changing goals can prompt dissatisfaction and a feeling of disappointment. To address this test, it's vital to set practical, reachable, and feasible objectives that line up with individual capacities and way of life.

Taking on a continuous way to deal with propensity development considers steady advancement. Instead of endeavoring to upgrade one's whole way of life short-term, center around making little, practical changes. When these works on become instilled propensities, extra changes can be presented. This bit by bit approach advances long haul accomplishment by staying balanced and disappointment.

Social impacts and outside tensions can likewise present difficulties in building sound propensities. Peer pressure, cultural assumptions, or clashing needs might affect individual decisions. Beating these outside impacts includes defining limits, conveying actually, and remaining consistent with individual qualities and needs.

Laying out transparent correspondence with people around you can assist with overseeing outside pressures. Obviously communicating individual wellbeing objectives, limits, and the significance of help can encourage understanding. Encircling oneself with similar people who share comparative wellbeing objectives can likewise give a strong local area, making it more straightforward to explore outer impacts.

Stress is an inescapable hindrance that can fundamentally influence the capacity to construct and support sound propensities. Persistent pressure can prompt close to home eating, upset rest, and a diminished inspiration for taking care of oneself. Successfully overseeing pressure is pivotal for generally speaking prosperity and propensity arrangement.

Integrating pressure the board methods into day to day schedules is fundamental. Practices like contemplation, profound breathing activities, or care can assist with lightening pressure. Normal actual work is likewise an intense pressure minimizer, delivering endorphins that further develop temperament and diminish strain. Understanding the wellsprings of stress and effectively attempting to address them, whether through critical thinking or looking for help, is urgent for long haul propensity arrangement.

Absence of help or a favorable climate is a critical obstruction to building solid propensities. Without a strong organization or a climate that encourages positive ways of behaving, people might find it trying to keep focused. Defeating this snag includes effectively looking for help, whether from companions, family, or local gatherings.

Conveying wellbeing objectives and the significance of help with those near you is an indispensable step. Participating in exercises with strong companions or relatives, for example, practicing together or getting ready good feasts collectively, can reinforce the feeling of local area. On the off chance that the current climate presents difficulties, think about rolling out purposeful improvements, for example, establishing a home climate that upholds smart dieting or finding new exercise spaces.

Absence of information or admittance to assets is one more snag that people might experience in their excursion to building sound propensities. Without the important data or instruments, arriving at informed conclusions about sustenance, exercise, and generally speaking prosperity becomes testing. Conquering this hindrance includes looking for solid data and using accessible assets.

Teaching oneself about sustenance, exercise, and wellbeing is a proactive move toward beating the hindrance of restricted information. Solid sources, like trustworthy sites, books, or counsels with medical care experts, can give important data. Using people group assets, for example, neighborhood wellness classes, studios, or care groups, can likewise improve admittance to information and backing.

In outline, addressing normal deterrents to building and supporting solid propensities requires a diverse methodology that considers the mental, ecological, and social parts of conduct change. Conquering difficulties, for example, absence of inspiration, time imperatives, moment delight, lingering, conflicting objective setting, social impacts, stress, absence of help, and restricted information includes executing functional techniques custom fitted to individual requirements.

These techniques incorporate interfacing wellbeing objectives to more profound inspirations, putting forth sensible and feasible objectives, overseeing time really, developing care, conquering delaying, defining limits, tending to outside pressures, overseeing pressure, looking for help, establishing a favorable climate, and procuring information. By getting it and proactively tending to these hindrances, people can explore the intricacies of propensity development and make enduring positive changes in their lives.

Conquering normal snags to building and supporting solid propensities is a nuanced and individualized process. Each challenge presents its own arrangement of intricacies, and tending to them requires a customized approach that considers mental, ecological, and conduct factors. In this investigation, we dig into commonsense methodologies to effectively beat pervasive obstructions, enabling people to explore the excursion of propensity arrangement.

1. **Absence of Inspiration:**
   Absence of inspiration is an unavoidable hindrance that can thwart progress in building solid propensities. To conquer this test, interfacing wellbeing objectives with natural motivations is significant. Dig profound to distinguish values that go past shallow cravings, for example, the longing to be available for friends and family or to improve by and large prosperity. Envisioning the drawn out advantages and understanding the individual meaning of wellbeing objectives can give a seriously getting through wellspring of inspiration.
   Useful Methodology: Set explicit, quantifiable, and attainable objectives, separating them into more modest, sensible advances. Praise every little triumph en route to support positive propensities and make a positive input circle, helping generally inspiration.
2. **Absence of Time:**
   Time imperatives frequently prevent people from participating in solid ways of behaving like activity, dinner arrangement, and taking care of oneself. To beat this hindrance, focus on and plan exercises purposely. Execute time usage methodologies, for example, making an everyday or week by week plan, to designate time for work out, dinner arranging, and other wellbeing related exercises.
   Viable Technique: Integrate actual work into everyday schedules, like using the stairwell rather than the lift or taking a stroll during breaks. Consolidate exercises, like associating while at the same time practicing or getting ready feasts in clusters, to augment accessible time.

3. **Moment Satisfaction versus Long haul Advantages:**
   The appeal of moment satisfaction over long haul advantages can make it trying to settle on better other options. To address this, shift the concentration from momentary compensations to long haul prosperity. Develop care to be available at the time and pursue cognizant decisions that line up with wellbeing objectives.
   Useful Technique: Practice careful eating by enjoying each nibble and focusing on craving and completion signals. Consider the drawn out results of decisions, settling on choices that add to in general wellbeing as opposed to looking for sure fire joy.
4. **Delaying:**
   Delaying is a typical obstacle that can obstruct the commencement of new propensities. To defeat this impediment, separate assignments into more modest, more sensible advances. Make a nitty gritty arrangement, set cut-off times, and use instruments like plans for the day or propensity following applications to give design and responsibility.
   Useful Technique: Look for help from companions, family, or wellbeing experts to give support and help with conquering lingering. Laying out an emotionally supportive network can offer inspiration and responsibility.
5. **Conflicting or Unreasonable Objective Setting:**
   Laying out excessively aggressive objectives or continually changing goals can prompt disappointment and a feeling of disappointment. Defeat this deterrent by setting reasonable, reachable, and feasible objectives that line up with individual capacities and way of life.
   Reasonable Procedure: Take on a progressive way to deal with propensity development, zeroing in on making little, feasible changes. Celebrate little triumphs, and when these works on become propensities, present extra changes.
6. **Social Impacts and Outer Tensions:**
   Peer pressure, cultural assumptions, or clashing needs might influence individual decisions. Beating outer impacts includes defining limits, conveying actually, and remaining consistent with individual qualities and needs.
   Down to earth System: Lay out transparent correspondence with everyone around you. Obviously express private wellbeing objectives and the significance of help. Encircle yourself with similar people who share comparative wellbeing objectives to make a steady local area.
7. **Stress:**
   Persistent pressure can fundamentally influence the capacity to construct and support solid propensities. Successfully overseeing pressure is vital for generally prosperity and propensity arrangement.
   Commonsense Procedure: Integrate pressure the executives strategies into

everyday schedules, like reflection, profound breathing activities, or care. Take part in standard active work, which discharges endorphins that further develop mind-set and lessen pressure. Address the wellsprings of stress through critical thinking or looking for help.

8. **Absence of Help or Favorable Climate:**
Without a steady organization or a climate that encourages positive ways of behaving, people might find it trying to remain focused. Beating this hindrance includes effectively looking for help, defining limits, and establishing a steady climate.

Reasonable Technique: Convey wellbeing objectives and the significance of help with those near you. Take part in exercises with strong companions or relatives. Assuming the current climate presents difficulties, think about rolling out deliberate improvements to establish a home climate that upholds solid propensities.

9. **Absence of Information or Admittance to Assets:**

Restricted information or admittance to assets can obstruct informed dynamic about sustenance, exercise, and generally speaking prosperity.

Useful Procedure: Teach oneself about sustenance, exercise, and wellbeing through solid sources like trustworthy sites, books, or discussions with medical care experts. Use people group assets, for example, neighborhood wellness classes, studios, or care groups, to upgrade admittance to information and backing.

In exploring the excursion of propensity arrangement, it's urgent to perceive that impediments are not outlandish road obstructions but rather difficulties to be tended to in a calculated way. Fitting these useful methodologies to individual requirements and conditions takes into consideration a more customized and viable methodology. As people develop flexibility, mindfulness, and a pledge to consistent improvement, they enable themselves to defeat impediments and fabricate reasonable, solid propensities for a satisfying life.

Chapter 8

Social Connections

Social associations are crucial parts of human existence, forming our encounters, feelings, and feeling of character. From the earliest transformative phases, people look for association with others, shaping bonds that impact their prosperity and social reconciliation. The multifaceted trap of social connections we develop all through our lives assumes a urgent part in forming our points of view, ways of behaving, and generally speaking personal satisfaction.

At the core of social associations is the nuclear family, frequently thought to be the foundation of human culture. Families give an establishment to daily reassurance, supporting, and the transmission of social qualities. The bonds framed inside families add to a singular's feeling of having a place and personality. Past the close family, more distant family individuals, like grandparents, aunties, and uncles, additionally assume significant parts in molding one's social associations.

As people progress through life, their groups of friends grow to incorporate companions, friends, and partners. Fellowships, specifically, hold a one of a kind importance in the social scene. Companions are much of the time picked in light of shared interests, values, and encounters, giving a feeling of kinship and common getting it. These associations add to close to home prosperity, offering support during testing times and commending victories.

In the advanced time, innovation has changed the scene of social associations. Web-based entertainment stages have become omnipresent, modifying the elements of how people assemble and keep up with connections. Online communications permit individuals to associate across geological limits, cultivating virtual networks in view of normal interests. While advanced associations can upgrade correspondence, they additionally bring up issues about the validness and profundity of these connections.

Social associations reach out past private connections to incorporate more extensive local area ties. Contribution in local area exercises, clubs, and associations cultivates a feeling of having a place and common perspective. Networks give a stage to joint effort, shared help, and aggregate critical thinking. Also, municipal commitment and volunteerism add to the general prosperity of the two people and the local area at large.

The work environment is one more critical field for social associations. Associates structure proficient connections that stretch out past the bounds of the workplace. Work environment associations impact work fulfillment, vocation advancement, and in general work insight. Cooperative endeavors and powerful correspondence inside a group add to a positive workplace, cultivating a feeling of local area and shared objectives.

As people explore the intricacies of social associations, they experience different difficulties. Struggle is an unavoidable part of connections, emerging from contrasts in sentiments, values, and assumptions. The capacity to explore and determine clashes is urgent for keeping up with sound associations. Successful correspondence, sympathy, and compromise assume imperative parts in tending to clashes and safeguarding connections.

Social associations additionally go through changes during significant life advances. Occasions like marriage, being a parent, or movement can reshape groups of friends and expect people to adjust to new elements. Keeping a harmony between existing connections and producing new ones is fundamental for exploring these changes effectively.

Dejection, then again, is an unavoidable test that can subvert the texture of social associations. Whether because of geological detachment, life conditions, or an absence of significant connections, depression can significantly affect mental and close to home prosperity. Addressing depression requires purposeful endeavors to construct and fortify social associations, underlining higher expectations when in doubt.

Social and cultural variables impact the idea of social associations. Social standards shape the assumptions and elements of connections, characterizing adequate types of social cooperation. Cultural designs, like monetary frameworks and social progressive systems, can affect the availability of social associations and impact the idea of relational connections.

The effect of social associations reaches out past individual prosperity to more extensive cultural results. Solid social securities add to social union and strength, cultivating a feeling of local area and shared character. Socially associated networks are better prepared to address difficulties, advance inclusivity, and establish strong conditions for people.

In any case, cultural patterns, like urbanization and the computerized age, have additionally acquainted difficulties with customary types of social associations. Metropolitan living, with its speedy way of life and transient nature, can add to social separation and a feeling of disengagement. The computerized age, while empowering virtual associations, has raised worries about the nature of these connections and their effect on eye to eye cooperations.

The idea of social capital exemplifies that social associations have substantial advantages for people and networks. Social capital alludes to the assets, both substantial and elusive, that emerge from connections and informal organizations. Trust, correspondence, and shared standards are fundamental parts of social capital, adding to the general prosperity and strength of networks.

One region where the significance of social associations is especially apparent is in emotional wellness. Solid social help has been connected to bring down paces of emotional well-being problems, expanded strength, and further developed survival techniques. On the other hand, social detachment and an absence of significant associations are risk factors for psychological wellness challenges, featuring the interconnectedness of social prosperity and mental wellbeing.

The formative meaning of social associations is apparent from youth. Connection hypothesis, proposed by John Bowlby, underlines the significance of secure connections in outset for solid profound and social turn of events. Kids who structure secure connections with guardians are bound to foster positive social connections and profound guideline abilities further down the road.

As people progress through puberty, peer connections accept more prominent significance. Peer impact can influence conduct, values, and personality during this formative stage. Positive companion connections add to social skill, while negative friend cooperations might prompt issues, for example, peer strain and social rejection.

The effect of social associations on actual wellbeing is a blossoming area of exploration. Studies have shown that people with strong informal communities experience better in general wellbeing results.

Social help has been connected to bring down death rates, worked on cardiovascular wellbeing, and upgraded safe capability. The instruments through which social associations impact actual wellbeing include both mental and physiological pathways.

Social associations assume a significant part in the maturing system, impacting the wellbeing and prosperity of more seasoned grown-ups. Dejection and social disengagement among the old are related with antagonistic wellbeing results, including expanded hazard of ongoing circumstances and mental degradation. Keeping up with social commitment and encouraging groups of people is fundamental for advancing solid maturing and moderating the pessimistic impacts of social separation.

In the domain of training, social associations are necessary to the growth opportunity. Peer communications, cooperative learning, and positive educator understudy connections add to scholastic achievement and socio-close to home turn of events. Schools act as significant social conditions where youngsters and youths acquire scholastic abilities as well as vital interactive abilities that shape their future connections.

The job of social associations in molding character is complex. Social and social affiliations add to the development of individual personality, affecting convictions, values, and self-discernment. Collaborations inside gatherings, like family, friends, and networks, give a setting to people to investigate and characterize their personalities. The exchange of character go on over the course of life, with social associations filling in as the two mirrors and forming powers.

With regards to close connections, social associations take on a particular aspect. Personal associations include the converging of individual lives, values, and desires. The nature of heartfelt connections is affected by successful correspondence, common comprehension, and shared objectives. Moreover, the more extensive social setting, including social standards and cultural assumptions, can affect the elements of heartfelt associations.

The elements of social associations are not insusceptible to the impact of more extensive social issues, including disparity and separation. Underlying imbalances in view of variables like race, orientation, and financial status can shape the nature and openness of social associations. Segregation and underestimation can prompt social prohibition, affecting people's capacity to shape significant associations and take part completely in the public arena.

The computerized time has introduced another period of social cooperations, portrayed by the predominance of online correspondence and virtual networks. Virtual entertainment stages, informing applications, and online discussions offer extraordinary open doors for association, permitting people to worldwide connect with others. Notwithstanding, the effect of computerized associations on the nature of connections and social prosperity is a subject of progressing banter.

While advanced associations can work with correspondence and the trading of thoughts, they additionally present difficulties. The arranged idea of online characters and the pervasiveness of social correlation can add to deep-seated insecurities and social nervousness. Moreover, the prompt idea of advanced correspondence might affect the profundity and realness of connections, bringing up issues about the real essence of online associations.

The idea of "FOMO" (apprehension about passing up a major opportunity) has arisen in the computerized age, featuring the uneasiness people might feel while seeing that others are partaking in remunerating encounters without them. This dread can be exacerbated by consistent openness to the exercises and accomplishments of others via online entertainment stages. Dealing with the mental effect of computerized associations requires care and a decent way to deal with online cooperations.

In spite of the difficulties presented by the advanced period, innovation additionally offers creative answers for encourage social associations. Virtual care groups, online networks, and telehealth administrations have become significant assets, particularly in the midst of physical separating and worldwide emergencies. The critical lies in utilizing innovation to supplement, as opposed to supplant, up close and personal cooperations and certified associations.

All in all, social associations structure the texture of human experience, impacting each part of life from outset to advanced age. The mind boggling snare of connections, incorporating family, companions, partners, and networks, shapes our personality, prosperity, and feeling of having a place. As people explore the difficulties of contention, advances, and depression, the nature of social associations becomes fundamental.

Cultural variables, including social standards and underlying disparities, impact the availability and nature of social associations. The computerized age has acquainted new aspects with social collaborations, bringing up issues about the credibility of online connections and their effect on prosperity. Be that as it may, innovation additionally presents potential chances to conquer actual obstructions and cultivate associations in imaginative ways.

Understanding the meaning of social associations is significant for people, networks, and social orders all in all. Sustaining and keeping up with positive connections add to mental, close to home, and actual prosperity. In an interconnected world, the capacity to explore the intricacies of social associations with sympathy, compelling correspondence, and a feeling of shared humankind is fundamental for encouraging a flourishing and strong worldwide local area.

8.1 Emphasizing the role of social relationships in health

The crossing point between friendly connections and wellbeing is a mind boggling and dynamic field that has earned expanding consideration from specialists, medical services experts, and policymakers. The acknowledgment that our associations with others can significantly affect our physical and mental prosperity has prompted a change in perspective by they way we comprehend and move toward medical care.

In this investigation, we dig into the many-sided manners by which social connections impact wellbeing results across the life expectancy, looking at the hidden systems, the job of different connections, and the ramifications for general wellbeing.

At the center of this request is the idea of social determinants of wellbeing, a system that recognizes the social, monetary, and ecological elements impacting wellbeing results. Social connections arise as a focal part of these determinants, applying an inescapable impact on people's wellbeing from youth to advanced age. The mind boggling exchange between friendly ties and wellbeing results is obvious in different areas, enveloping actual wellbeing, mental prosperity, and even mortality.

Beginning with the early stages of life, the effect of social connections on well-being starts to come to fruition. In earliest stages, the nature of parental figure kid collaborations establishes the groundwork for close to home turn of events and connection. Connection hypothesis, spearheaded by John Bowlby, places that protected connections in youth are pivotal for the improvement of trust, profound guideline, and the development of sound connections further down the road. Babies who experience predictable and responsive providing care are bound to foster secure connection designs, encouraging a feeling of safety that stretches out to future social connections.

As youngsters progress through youth, peer connections expect expanding importance. Peer cooperations add to social and close to home turn of events, impacting ways of behaving, mentalities, and survival strategies. Positive companion connections offer a help framework during the difficulties of youthfulness, adding to flexibility and mental prosperity. On the other hand, negative friend encounters, like tormenting or social avoidance, can unfavorably affect psychological well-being, featuring the basic job of social connections in molding the juvenile experience.

Relational peculiarities, one more essential component of social connections, keep on assuming a critical part in wellbeing results all through the life expectancy. The nuclear family fills in as an essential wellspring of consistent encouragement, forming people's impression of self and others. Sound family connections add to a positive socio-close to home climate, cultivating a feeling of having a place and security. Conversely, broken relational peculiarities, described by struggle or disregard, can add to pressure and adversely influence both mental and actual wellbeing.

The impact of social connections on wellbeing stretches out into adulthood and is especially articulated with regards to heartfelt associations. Close connections, described by profound closeness and shared help, have been connected to various medical advantages. Hitched people, for instance, will quite often display lower death rates and better in general wellbeing contrasted with their unmarried partners.

The basic reassurance gave inside heartfelt associations can cushion against pressure, add to cardiovascular wellbeing, and improve by and large prosperity.

Companionships, frequently depicted as picked relatives, likewise assume a fundamental part in grown-up friendly associations. The nature of kinships has been related with emotional wellness, life fulfillment, and even life span. Companions offer profound help, friendship, and a feeling of having a place. The social exercises and shared encounters inside companionships add to a satisfying and improved life, building up the possibility that the expansiveness and profundity of social associations matter for wellbeing results.

Prescription For A Healthy Life

In the work environment, social connections take on a special aspect. Associates and expert organizations impact work fulfillment, feelings of anxiety, and generally speaking work insight. Positive working environment connections add to a strong and cooperative workplace, cultivating a feeling of having a place and shared objectives. Alternately, work environment stressors and harmful relational elements can antagonistically affect psychological well-being and add to burnout.

Past individual connections, local area associations structure one more layer of the social determinants of wellbeing. Inclusion in local area exercises, metro commitment, and a feeling of having a place with a bigger aggregate add to in general prosperity. Networks that focus on friendly attachment, encouraging groups of people, and inclusivity will generally display better wellbeing results. The accessibility of local area assets, like parks, sporting offices, and medical care administrations, additionally shapes the wellbeing scene of a local area.

The effect of social connections on wellbeing isn't restricted to mental and close to home prosperity; it reaches out to actual wellbeing results too. Research has reliably exhibited the connection between solid social ties and lower paces of persistent sicknesses. Cardiovascular wellbeing, specifically, is impacted by the nature of social associations. People with powerful interpersonal organizations have been displayed to have lower circulatory strain, decreased chance of coronary illness, and better cardiovascular results.

The components through which social connections influence actual wellbeing are different and interconnected. One key pathway includes the impact of social associations on wellbeing ways of behaving. Solid ways of behaving, like standard activity, adjusted nourishment, and adherence to clinical suggestions, are in many cases built up inside informal communities. On the other hand, social seclusion or negative connections might add to undesirable ways of behaving, like unfortunate dietary decisions, stationary ways of life, and resistance with clinical counsel.

The pressure buffering speculation gives one more focal point through which to figure out the connection between friendly associations and wellbeing. Social help goes about as a support against the physiological and mental impacts of pressure.

People areas of strength for with emotionally supportive networks might encounter lower levels of pressure chemicals, better safe capability, and quicker recuperation from unpleasant circumstances. The basic reassurance given by friendly connections adds to a feeling that all is well with the world and strength notwithstanding life's difficulties.

The impact of social connections on wellbeing results is especially notable with regards to emotional well-being. Various investigations have laid out a strong relationship between friendly associations and mental prosperity. Social help fills in as a defensive component against the improvement of psychological well-being problems and adds to recuperation for people encountering emotional well-being difficulties.

Depression, described by an apparent absence of significant social associations, has arisen as a critical gamble factor for emotional wellness issues. The abstract insight of dejection is particular from social disengagement; an individual can feel forlorn in any event, when encircled by others. Tireless dejection has been connected to expanded paces of despondency, uneasiness, and mental degradation. Perceiving the effect of dejection on emotional wellness highlights the significance of developing and keeping up with significant social connections.

The impact of social connections on emotional well-being is apparent across the life expectancy. In youth and puberty, positive social cooperations add to the advancement of interactive abilities, profound guideline, and versatility. Peer connections assume a vital part in molding confidence and character during these early stages. Alternately, encounters of social prohibition or tormenting can lastingly affect psychological well-being, highlighting the weakness of people during this formative stage.

In adulthood, the job of social connections in emotional well-being becomes entwined with the complicated requests of work, family, and cultural assumptions. Adjusting contending liabilities and keeping up with social associations can be testing, especially notwithstanding life advances, for example, being a parent, vocation changes, or movement. Compelling survival methods and a powerful emotionally supportive network are fundamental for exploring the stressors of adulthood while saving mental prosperity.

More seasoned grown-ups, confronting one of a kind difficulties like retirement, loss of friends and family, and potential medical problems, get critical advantages from social associations. Social commitment among more established grown-ups is related with worked on mental capability, diminished chance of sorrow, and expanded life fulfillment. Keeping up with informal organizations in late life adds to sound maturing and mitigates the adverse consequences of social confinement, which is a common issue among the older.

The ramifications of the connection between friendly associations and wellbeing are sweeping, stretching out past the person to more extensive cultural results. Solid social securities add to social union, local area strength, and a feeling of aggregate personality.

Networks portrayed by steady informal communities are better prepared to address general wellbeing challenges, answer emergencies, and advance by and large prosperity.

Notwithstanding, cultural patterns and changes in social standards have acquainted difficulties with customary types of social associations. Urbanization, with its speedy way of life and accentuation on independence, can add to social segregation and a feeling of separation. The computerized age, while working with virtual associations, has brought up issues about the nature of these connections and their effect on eye to eye communications.

8.2 Discussing the impact of loneliness and isolation

The effect of forlornness and confinement on people is an intricate and inescapable part of the human experience that reaches out across different life stages. Depression, frequently characterized as the emotional sensation of social confinement or an absence of significant associations, can have significant ramifications for both mental and actual prosperity. Confinement, then again, alludes to the goal condition actually isolated from others. While these ideas are particular, they frequently coincide, and the interaction among depression and separation can worsen their individual impacts. In this investigation, we dig into the multi-layered ramifications of dejection and disengagement, looking at their consequences for psychological wellness, actual wellbeing, and more extensive cultural results.

Dejection isn't simply a transient profound state yet an industrious and inescapable condition that can lastingly affect psychological wellness. The emotional idea of depression makes it a profoundly private encounter, and people might feel forlorn in any event, when encircled by others. The wellsprings of depression are assorted and can come from social, mental, or ecological elements. For instance, people encountering significant life changes like migration, retirement, or the departure of a friend or family member might be especially helpless to sensations of depression.

The effect of depression on emotional wellness is apparent across the life expectancy, from youth to advanced age. In youngsters and youths, dejection can add to a scope of mental difficulties, including sorrow, uneasiness, and low confidence. Peer connections assume a urgent part during these early stages, and encounters of social rejection or harassing can leave enduring profound scars. Tending to dejection in youthful people is fundamental for advancing sound socio-close to home turn of events and forestalling the beginning of emotional well-being problems.

During adulthood, the difficulties related with forlornness might heighten as people explore the intricacies of work, connections, and cultural assumptions. The requests of profession, life as a parent, and different obligations can make hindrances to social association, prompting expanded weakness to dejection.

The computerized age, while offering valuable open doors for virtual association, has additionally been ensnared in the ascent of social detachment and depression, as online cooperations may not completely substitute for up close and personal connections.

In more seasoned grown-ups, the effect of forlornness on psychological wellbeing is especially articulated. Maturing is frequently joined by life changes like retirement, loss of companions or relatives, and potential medical problems, all of which can add to social disengagement and sensations of forlornness. The pervasiveness of dejection among more established grown-ups is a critical general wellbeing concern, given its relationship with mental degradation, sorrow, and an expanded gamble of mortality. Tending to depression in the old is vital for advancing solid maturing and improving generally speaking prosperity.

The mental results of forlornness stretch out past individual prosperity to cultural results. Depression has been connected to diminished municipal commitment, decreased trust in others, and a lessened feeling of local area. In social orders where social associations are debilitated, people might feel less put resources into aggregate prosperity, adding to a feeling of social discontinuity. Tending to the cultural ramifications of depression requires an all encompassing methodology that joins individual intercessions with more extensive local area and strategy measures.

While depression is an emotional close to home state, seclusion alludes to the goal state of being truly isolated from others. Detachment can happen because of different variables, including geological distance, actual inability, or systematization. The objective idea of disconnection frequently intensifies the emotional experience of depression, causing what is going on where people feel socially secluded as well as actually isolated from significant social communications.

One of the most pervasive types of detachment is social segregation, which happens when people have restricted contact with family, companions, or local area. Social separation can result from variables like living alone, absence of transportation, or actual wellbeing impediments that confine versatility. The outcomes of social confinement are extensive, influencing mental and actual wellbeing, as well as in general personal satisfaction. More seasoned grown-ups, specifically, are helpless against social segregation, particularly on the off chance that they experience loss of versatility, deprivation, or live in long haul care offices.

The actual wellbeing ramifications of detachment are significant and multi-layered. Socially segregated people are at an expanded gamble of creating constant circumstances like cardiovascular illness, hypertension, and corpulence. The physiological instruments connecting separation to chronic weakness results include the dysregulation of stress chemicals, aggravation, and compromised safe capability. The effect of segregation on cardiovascular wellbeing, specifically, is imperative, with research showing that socially secluded people have a higher gamble of coronary illness and stroke.

Moreover, confinement has been related with hindering wellbeing ways of behaving, including unfortunate nourishment, stationary ways of life, and non-adherence to clinical exhortation. The absence of social help might add to a decrease in taking care of oneself works on, compounding existing medical issue and obstructing recuperation from sickness. Perceiving the interconnectedness of social associations and actual wellbeing is fundamental for creating extensive medical care techniques that address both the mental and physiological parts of prosperity.

Separation likewise has significant ramifications for psychological well-being, frequently interlacing with the experience of dejection. The shortfall of significant social associations can add to sensations of despondency, sadness, and tension. The mental cost of detachment is apparent in different populaces, remembering detainees for isolation, people with restricted admittance to social help, and those encountering long haul organization.

With regards to the computerized age, virtual associations and online cooperations might offer a similarity to social commitment, yet they may not completely substitute for eye to eye connections. The nature of social collaborations is vital, and the shortfall of in-person associations can add to a feeling of detachment and estrangement. Furthermore, the pervasiveness of advanced correspondence doesn't dispense with the gamble of actual disconnection, as people might in any case need significant in-person communications.

The effect of disengagement on emotional wellness is especially notable among weak populaces, like people with inabilities or persistent ailments. Restricted portability or availability issues might add to actual disconnection, limiting people's capacity to partake in friendly exercises and draw in with their networks. The psychosocial results of confinement in these populaces can be significant, influencing generally speaking life fulfillment and mental prosperity.

In the working environment, disengagement can appear as friendly or expert separation, the two of which have suggestions for individual and authoritative results. Social segregation at work, portrayed by an absence of significant connections with partners, can add to sensations of estrangement and occupation disappointment. Proficient disconnection, then again, may result from an absence of mentorship, cooperation, or acknowledgment inside the working environment, influencing vocation improvement and occupation execution.

The ramifications of forlornness and confinement stretch out past the person to more extensive cultural difficulties. As social orders wrestle with the outcomes of social fracture, policymakers and networks should consider the financial and medical care loads related with these issues. The expense of tending to mental and actual wellbeing challenges originating from dejection and disengagement highlights the significance of protection measures and exhaustive social arrangements.

Tending to dejection and disengagement requires a diverse methodology that incorporates individual, local area, and strategy level intercessions. At the singular level, cultivating familiarity with the significance of social associations and giving assets to building and it is fundamental to keep up with connections. Instructive projects that advance interactive abilities, compassion, and viable correspondence can add to a culture that qualities and focuses on human associations.

Local area based drives assume an essential part in tending to depression and seclusion. Making social spaces, coordinating local area occasions, and executing programs that work with intergenerational communications add to building a feeling of having a place and shared character. Besides, people group encouraging groups of people, including neighborhood affiliations, strict foundations, and non-benefit associations, can assume a vital part in recognizing and supporting people in danger of depression and separation.

According to a strategy viewpoint, tending to forlornness and confinement requires an organized exertion that traverses medical care, social administrations, and local area improvement. Incorporating social determinants of wellbeing into medical services strategies and practices is fundamental for perceiving and tending to the psychosocial parts of prosperity. Also, strategies that focus on reasonable lodging, available transportation, and local area framework add to establishing conditions that cultivate social associations.

With regards to maturing populaces, approaches that help sound maturing and age-accommodating networks are pivotal. Advancing drives that empower more established grown-ups to stay dynamic, drew in, and associated with their networks mitigates the gamble of social detachment.

8.3 Providing strategies for building and maintaining meaningful connections

Constructing and keeping up with significant associations is a deep rooted try that adds to the extravagance and satisfaction of human existence. In a period described by mechanical headways, speedy ways of life, and cultural changes, the significance of purposeful endeavors to encourage veritable connections couldn't possibly be more significant. In this investigation, we dig into methodologies for building and keeping up with significant associations across different settings, including family, companionships, heartfelt connections, work environment collaborations, and local area commitment.

Family Associations:

The nuclear family fills in as the fundamental structure block of social associations. Sustaining and keeping up with significant family connections add to a feeling of having a place, everyday reassurance, and shared character. Transparent correspondence shapes the bedrock of solid family associations. Customary discussions, undivided attention, and the declaration of sentiments assist with cultivating common comprehension and trust inside the family.

Quality time spent together is instrumental in building solid family bonds. Taking part in shared exercises, whether it be family feasts, trips, or side interests, sets out open doors for association and supports a feeling of harmony. Also, praising achievements, recognizing accomplishments, and offering profound help during testing times fortify family ties.

Laying out and keeping up with family customs is one more remarkable procedure for building associations. Customs and schedules, whether they include special festivals, week after week suppers, or yearly excursions, make a feeling of progression and shared history. These customs act as standards that tight spot relatives together and add to a feeling of personality and having a place.

Companionship Associations:

Prescription For A Healthy Life

Fellowships assume a novel and significant part in our lives, offering friendship, support, and shared encounters. Constructing and keeping up with significant kinships require purposeful endeavors and a veritable interest in the prosperity of one another. Starting and responding thoughtful gestures, whether large or little, cultivates a feeling of common consideration and fortifies the underpinning of kinship.

Viable correspondence is a foundation of significant companionships. Sharing considerations, sentiments, and encounters advances understanding and association. Past superficial discussions, digging into additional significant points and being open to each other extends the connection between companions. Undivided attention, compassion, and approval add to establishing a climate of trust and receptiveness.

Consistency and dependability are key components in keeping up with fellowships. Being reliable and accessible when required forms trust and consoles companions that they can depend on one another. Normal registrations, whether through calls, messages, or in-person gatherings, show a continuous obligation to the fellowship and assist with forestalling sensations of disregard or seclusion.

Shared exercises and interests structure the premise of numerous fellowships. Taking part in side interests, sports, or imaginative pursuits together gives a stage to divided happiness and reinforces the association among companions. Partaking in one another's lives, whether by going to occasions, praising accomplishments, or offering help during difficulties, builds up the feeling of fellowship.

Heartfelt Associations:

Close connections bring an exceptional arrangement of elements and require deliberate endeavors to construct and support significant associations. Correspondence is principal in heartfelt organizations. Communicating sentiments, requirements, and assumptions straightforwardly and consciously encourages a more profound comprehension between accomplices. Customary and fair correspondence makes an underpinning of trust and close to home closeness.

Quality time spent together is fundamental for the wellbeing of close connections. In the midst of occupied plans, cutting out time for shared exercises, date evenings, or basically calm minutes reinforces the connection between accomplices. Making ceremonies and schedules inside the relationship, like week by week meals or end of the week escapes, gives potential open doors to association and builds up the feeling of responsibility.

Exploring difficulties together is a fundamental piece of building major areas of strength for an association. Struggle is unavoidable, however moving toward conflicts with compassion, undivided attention, and a cooperative mentality encourages a feeling of collaboration. Figuring out how to think twice about, shared conviction, and finding productive arrangements add to the flexibility of the relationship.

Individual development and independence are fundamental inside heartfelt associations. Supporting each other's very own objectives, interests, and yearnings makes a good overall arrangement among fellowship and individual satisfaction. Empowering self-improvement and commending each other's accomplishments add to a flourishing and steady heartfelt organization.

Work environment Associations:

Constructing and keeping up with significant associations in the work environment is vital for a positive and cooperative workplace. Compelling correspondence is central in proficient connections. Clear and open correspondence, whether in group gatherings, one-on-one connections, or composed correspondences, cultivates understanding and advances a culture of straightforwardness.

Coordinated effort and collaboration add to the strength of working environment associations. Empowering a cooperative outlook, perceiving and esteeming different viewpoints, and encouraging a culture of common help establish a positive workplace. Shared objectives and a feeling of aggregate reason upgrade the association between partners.

Acknowledgment and appreciation are useful assets in building work environment associations. Recognizing and praising individual and group accomplishments, offering thanks, and giving positive input add to a culture of regard and fellowship. Feeling esteemed and valued cultivates a feeling of association and obligation to the working environment.

Social exercises and group building practices outside the extent of normal work errands can add to building significant associations in the work environment. Sorting out group occasions, withdraws, or easygoing social events gives an open door to partners to cooperate in a more casual environment, encouraging connections past the limits of the workplace.

Local area Associations:

Drawing in with the more extensive local area is a fundamental part of building significant associations and adding to the prosperity of society. Chipping in and local area administration furnish chances to associate with other people who share comparative qualities and a promise to having a beneficial outcome. Co-operating towards a shared objective cultivates a feeling of local area and mutual perspective.

Taking part in local area occasions and exercises assists people with turning out to be more coordinated into the social texture of their environmental elements. Going to nearby get-togethers, widespread developments, or neighborhood gatherings gives chances to meet new individuals, structure associations, and add to the dynamic quality of the local area. Shared encounters make a feeling of having a place.

Supporting neighborhood drives and organizations is a substantial method for building associations inside the local area. Whether through shopping locally, taking part in local area tasks, or going to municipal events, people add to the strength and versatility of the local area. Shared interests in neighborhood organizations make a feeling of interconnectedness.

Systems administration and coordinated effort with similar people or associations can be instrumental in building significant associations at the local area level. Joining clubs, affiliations, or backing bunches permits people to associate with other people who share normal interests, objectives, or values. These associations add to a feeling of shared character and reason inside the local area.

Advanced Associations:

In the advanced age, innovation gives new roads to building and keeping up with associations. While online cooperations can be important, they ought to supplement as opposed to supplant up close and personal associations. Using web-based entertainment stages, online networks, and informing applications can work with correspondence and assist people with remaining associated with companions, family, and networks.

Careful advanced correspondence is fundamental for building significant associations on the web. Participating in significant discussions, communicating veritable interest, and effectively partaking in virtual networks add to the genuineness of computerized associations. Being deliberate about the substance shared and consumed establishes a positive web-based climate.

Adjusting computerized cooperations with disconnected associations is significant for generally prosperity. While online associations can give comfort and availability, eye to eye connections stay principal to building profound and significant connections. Dispensing time for face to face gatherings, calls, or different types of direct correspondence adds to a more all encompassing and satisfying public activity.

Self-Reflection and Self-improvement:

Fabricating and keeping up with significant associations likewise require a level of mindfulness and self-improvement. Taking part in self-reflection permits people to figure out their own requirements, values, and correspondence styles. Realizing oneself adds to more credible and satisfying associations with others.

Developing characteristics like sympathy, empathy, and undivided attention improves the nature of associations. Being sensitive to the feelings and encounters of others cultivates a more profound comprehension and association. Furthermore, rehearsing graciousness and liberality adds to establishing a positive and steady friendly climate.

Constant self-improvement and learning add to the lavishness of associations. Being available to new encounters, points of view, and thoughts expands' comprehension one might interpret the world and takes into account more different and significant associations.

Keeping up with significant associations is a deep rooted pursuit that assumes an essential part in molding the nature of our lives. Whether with regards to family, kinships, close connections, working environment cooperations, or local area commitment, the capacity to support and support profound, genuine associations is fundamental for close to home prosperity, self-improvement, and cultural agreement. In this investigation, we dig into the complex methodologies and rules that add to keeping up with significant associations across different circles of life.

1. **Correspondence:**
Compelling correspondence shapes the bedrock of every significant association. It includes articulating one's thoughts as well as effectively paying attention to other people. In relational peculiarities, transparent correspondence cultivates understanding and reinforces bonds. In companionships, the capacity to share considerations, sentiments, and encounters develops the association. In heartfelt connections, correspondence is the foundation of profound closeness. At work, clear and straightforward correspondence is significant for cooperation and collaboration. Inside people group, correspondence fabricates spans and works with understanding.

Correspondence likewise stretches out to the computerized domain, where the smart utilization of innovation can improve associations. In any case, it's crucial for find some kind of harmony, guaranteeing that virtual cooperations supplement, as opposed to supplant, up close and personal correspondence. Careful and sympathetic correspondence establishes the groundwork for trust, weakness, and a common perspective, cultivating getting through associations.

2. **Quality Time:**
Focusing on connections is an unmistakable articulation of responsibility and prioritization. In familial bonds, hanging out fortifies the feeling of having a place. In kinships, shared exercises and encounters make enduring recollections.

In heartfelt connections, cutting out time for one another encourages profound closeness. Inside the working environment, shared projects and cooperative endeavors extend proficient associations. In people group, partaking in nearby occasions and exercises constructs a feeling of shared character.

The idea of value time isn't just about amount yet in addition about the goal and presence during those minutes. Significant associations are developed when people are completely drawn in, effectively taking part, and exhibiting a real interest in the prosperity of others. Whether through shared leisure activities, dinners, or straightforward discussions, the speculation of time sustains associations.

3. **Compassion and Understanding:**
   Sympathy, the capacity to comprehend and discuss the thoughts of another, is a foundation of significant associations. It includes venturing into the shoes of others, perceiving their points of view, and answering with empathy. In family connections, sympathy cultivates basic reassurance during testing times. In kinships, it makes a space for weakness and shared understanding. In heartfelt connections, compassion constructs an underpinning of profound closeness. At work, understanding partners' points of view advances a positive workplace. Inside people group, sympathy fortifies the texture of shared encounters.
   Developing sympathy requires undivided attention, the capacity to keep judgment, and a certified interest in others' encounters. It includes recognizing and approving the feelings of those we interface with. By rehearsing sympathy, people add to making a strong and grasping social biological system.

4. **Shared Values and Objectives:**
   Significant associations are in many cases established in shared values, convictions, or shared objectives. In familial bonds, shared values add to a feeling of solidarity and shared personality. In companionships, normal interests structure the premise of association. In heartfelt connections, adjusting life objectives reinforces the organization. Inside the work environment, a common hierarchical mission encourages a feeling of direction. In people group, shared values add to a durable and agreeable social texture.
   Distinguishing and sustaining shared values includes open and progressing discussions. It requires a shared investigation of what makes the biggest difference to people and how those values adjust. Laying out shared conviction gives an internal compass and motivation, building up the associations that are based upon a groundwork of shared values.

5. **Trust and Weakness:**
   Trust is a central component of significant associations. It includes a confidence in the dependability, honesty, and validness of others. In family connections, trust is the magic that binds the unit. In kinships, trust considers weakness and receptiveness.
   In close connections, trust frames the premise of profound closeness. In the working environment, trust is fundamental for compelling coordinated effort. In people group, trust cultivates a feeling of safety and collaboration. Building trust requires consistency, unwavering quality, and an honorable exhibition over the long run. It likewise includes a readiness to be powerless. Weakness, the demonstration of opening oneself up inwardly, is complementary in significant associations. It establishes a climate where people have a

solid sense of reassurance to share their credible selves, cultivating a more profound comprehension and association.

6. **Versatility and Adaptability:**
Life is dynamic, and keeping up with significant associations requires versatility and adaptability. In relational peculiarities, adjusting to life changes guarantees the strength of associations. In companionships, adaptability considers the rhythmic movement of individual lives. In heartfelt connections, flexibility is vital for exploring changes together. At work, adaptability in jobs and obligations adds to a positive workplace. Inside people group, versatility considers development and advancement.

Being versatile includes a readiness to embrace change and explore difficulties together. It requires correspondence about advancing necessities and assumptions. Significant associations are supported when people can adjust to the unavoidable changes in life conditions without compromising the center underpinning of their connections.

7. **Appreciation and Appreciation:**
Offering thanks and appreciation reinforces the texture of significant associations. In family connections, recognizing the commitments of every part encourages a positive environment. In kinships, offering thanks for the help and friendship makes a complementary bond. In heartfelt connections, appreciating each other's characteristics upgrades the association. At work, perceiving partners' endeavors adds to a positive work culture. Inside people group, offering thanks fabricates a culture of common help.

Developing an act of appreciation includes consistently recognizing and communicating appreciation for the positive parts of connections. It tends to be basically as straightforward as communicating gratitude for an act of kindness or perceiving the characteristics that make every association unique. Appreciation supports positive associations and adds to a culture of benevolence.

8. **Limits and Independence:**
Keeping up with sound associations includes laying out and regarding limits. In family connections, clear limits add to shared regard. In kinships, understanding individual space and independence improves the association. In close connections, regarding each other's singularity encourages a feeling of organization.

At work, defining proficient limits adds to a positive workplace. Inside people group, perceiving and regarding individual limits guarantees an agreeable conjunction.

Laying out and imparting limits requires mindfulness and open discourse. It includes understanding individual requirements for independence and guaranteeing that those needs are regarded inside the setting of the relationship.

Sound associations flourish when there is a harmony among fellowship and individual space.

9. **Compromise:**
Struggle is a characteristic piece of any relationship, and significant associations are supported by compelling compromise. In relational peculiarities, tending to clashes transparently forestalls hatred. In kinships, exploring conflicts with deference reinforces the bond. In close connections, settling clashes encourages profound closeness. At work, tending to clashes advances a positive work culture. Inside people group, settling contrasts usefully guarantees social amicability.

Viable compromise includes undivided attention, sympathy, and a readiness to track down commonly gainful arrangements. It requires an emphasis on understanding the underlying drivers of contentions as opposed to finding fault. Significant associations are reinforced when people can explore clashes with deference, compassion, and a guarantee to tracking down goal.

10. **Self-awareness and Shared Encounters:**

Individual development adds to the lavishness of associations. In family connections, supporting each other's self-improvement reinforces the nuclear family. In companionships, celebrating individual accomplishments and achievements improves the association. In close connections, empowering each other's yearnings adds to a flourishing organization. At work, encouraging open doors for proficient development reinforces working environment associations. Inside people group, shared encounters and aggregate development add to a feeling of having a place.

Developing self-awareness includes a promise to continuous learning, self-reflection, and embracing new encounters. Significant associations are extended when people can share their singular processes and commend the development and accomplishments of those they interface with.

Chapter 9

Creating Your Personal Health Plan

In the hurrying around of current life, it's barely noticeable the significance of keeping a sound way of life. The requests of work, family, and different obligations frequently come first, allowing for taking care of oneself. Notwithstanding, putting time and exertion into making an individual wellbeing plan is vital for long haul prosperity. This far reaching guide means to assist you with fostering a customized wellbeing plan that incorporates physical, mental, and close to home perspectives, cultivating an all encompassing way to deal with your general health.

Surveying Your Ongoing Wellbeing Status

Prior to digging into the complexities of making an individual wellbeing plan, considering your ongoing wellbeing status is fundamental. Leading an intensive self-evaluation permits you to recognize regions that need improvement and sets the establishment for practical and reachable objectives. Start by assessing your actual wellbeing through a far reaching assessment of your eating regimen, work-out daily schedule, and rest designs.

Actual Wellbeing

Think about your dietary propensities and their effect on your general wellbeing. Observe the kinds of food varieties you routinely eat, focusing on the equilibrium of macronutrients and the consideration of fundamental nutrients and minerals. Survey whether your ongoing eating routine backings your energy levels, invulnerable framework, and long haul wellbeing objectives.

Then, assess your work-out everyday practice. Ponder the recurrence, force, and sort of proactive tasks you take part in consistently. Decide whether your ongoing activity routine lines up with your wellness objectives and advances cardiovascular wellbeing, strength, and adaptability.

In conclusion, dissect your rest designs. Satisfactory and quality rest is crucial to by and large prosperity. Consider your daily rest span, rest climate, and any potential elements influencing the nature of your rest. Perceiving regions for development in your rest routine is urgent for enhancing your actual wellbeing.

Mental and Profound Wellbeing

Moving past actual wellbeing, it's basic to survey your psychological and close to home prosperity. Ponder your feelings of anxiety, strategies for dealing with stress, and by and large close to home state. Consider the wellsprings of stress in your life, whether they are business related, individual, or natural. Perceive how you normally adapt to pressure and whether these components are solid and practical.

Also, assess your close to home strength and mindfulness. Observe your close to home triggers and how you answer testing circumstances. Creating the capacity to appreciate people on a profound level is fundamental for keeping up with mental and close to home equilibrium.

Putting forth Sensible and Attainable Objectives

Whenever you've surveyed your ongoing wellbeing status, the following stage is to put forth practical and reachable objectives. Laying out clear targets gives guidance and inspiration, assisting you with remaining fixed on your excursion to better wellbeing.

Actual Wellbeing Objectives

Regarding actual wellbeing, put forth unambiguous objectives for your eating regimen, exercise, and rest. For instance, on the off chance that you distinguish a need to work on your eating regimen, lay out quantifiable targets like integrating more products of the soil into your everyday dinners, decreasing the admission of handled food sources, or remaining hydrated by drinking a sufficient measure of water every day.

With regards to work out, put forth practical wellness objectives in light of your ongoing wellness level and wanted results. Whether it's rising the recurrence of your exercises, working on your perseverance, or dominating another active work, pick objectives that challenge you without overpowering your ability.

For rest, lay out a reliable rest plan and establish a favorable rest climate. Go for the gold number of long stretches of rest every evening and execute unwinding methods to work on the nature of your rest.

Mental and Close to home Wellbeing Objectives

In the domain of mental and profound wellbeing, consider defining objectives connected with pressure the board and close to home prosperity. This could include taking on care rehearses, like reflection or profound breathing activities, to develop a feeling of quiet and presence in your regular routine. Furthermore, put forth objectives for upgrading your capacity to understand people on a deeper level, for example, further developing relational abilities or looking for help from a specialist or guide when required.

Planning Your Customized Activity Plan

Considering clear objectives, now is the right time to plan a customized move plan that frames the particular advances you'll initiate to accomplish them. Your activity plan ought to be custom-made to your one of a kind requirements, inclinations, and way of life, it guaranteeing that is both down to earth and feasible.

Actual Wellbeing Activity Plan

Integrate changes to your eating routine steadily, zeroing in on little, manageable alterations. This could include feast preparing to guarantee better food decisions, step by step decreasing the admission of sweet or handled food sources, and being aware of part estimates. Consider talking with a nutritionist for customized direction in light of your dietary inclinations and wellbeing objectives.

For your work-out daily practice, plan a timetable that lines up with your way of life. Pick exercises that you appreciate to improve the probability of consistency. In the event that you're new to work out, begin with moderate-force exercises and slowly progress. Enroll the help of an exercise mate or consider employing a fitness coach for added inspiration and direction.

To work on your rest, lay out a sleep time schedule that signs to your body that now is the right time to slow down. This might incorporate exercises like perusing, rehearsing unwinding procedures, or staying away from electronic gadgets before sleep time. Establish an agreeable rest climate by putting resources into a quality bedding and pads and limiting clamor and light unsettling influences.

Mental and Close to home Wellbeing Activity Plan

Focus on pressure the board by integrating care rehearses into your everyday daily practice. This can be basically as straightforward as enjoying short reprieves over the course of the day to rehearse profound breathing or care contemplation. Distinguish exercises that give you pleasure and unwinding, whether it's investing energy in nature, taking part in a side interest, or associating with friends and family.

Upgrade your ability to understand people on a profound level through self-reflection and mindfulness works out. Journaling can be an important instrument for investigating your contemplations and feelings. Also, look for open doors for self-awareness, for example, going to studios or perusing writing that grows how you might interpret yourself as well as other people.

Executing Way of life Changes

Executing way of life changes requires responsibility and consistency. As you leave on your excursion to better wellbeing, be ready to experience difficulties and mishaps. Take on a development mentality that perspectives challenges as any open doors for learning and improvement.

Actual Wellbeing Way of life Changes

Consolidate your dietary changes bit by bit, exploring different avenues regarding new recipes and tracking down better options in contrast to your number one food sources. Consider signing up for a cooking class or investigating various foods to make the interaction charming. Remain aware of your dietary patterns, rehearsing instinctive eating to more readily comprehend your body's yearning and completion signals.

Focus on your work-out everyday practice by booking devoted exercise meetings in your schedule. Make actual work a non-debatable piece of your everyday practice, and be adaptable in adjusting your exercises to oblige changes in your timetable. Celebrate little wellness achievements, whether it's finishing a difficult exercise or working on your exhibition in a particular activity.

Develop sound rest propensities by making a loosening up sleep time schedule. Limit screen time before bed, establish a dull and calm rest climate, and go for the gold rest plan. On the off chance that rest unsettling influences endure, consider talking with a rest expert to recognize and resolve hidden issues.

Mental and Close to home Wellbeing Way of life Changes

Coordinate care rehearses into your everyday existence by integrating short contemplation meetings or care practices into your daily schedule. Use care to explore upsetting circumstances, zeroing in on the current second as opposed to becoming overpowered by future vulnerabilities. Develop a positive outlook by rehearsing appreciation and reexamining negative contemplations.

Sustain your ability to appreciate anyone at their core by effectively paying attention to other people and looking to figure out alternate points of view. Participate in transparent correspondence, offering your viewpoints and sentiments in a helpful way. Focus on taking care of oneself exercises that give you pleasure and unwinding, whether it's investing energy with friends and family, participating in imaginative pursuits, or just going for a relaxed stroll.

Checking Progress and Changing Your Arrangement

Consistently screen your advancement to guarantee that your own wellbeing plan stays successful and lined up with your objectives. Survey both quantitative and subjective parts of your prosperity to acquire a complete comprehension of your general wellbeing.

Actual Wellbeing Observing

Keep a food journal to follow your dietary decisions and recognize examples or regions for development. Screen your energy levels, mind-set, and any actual changes as you make adjustments to your eating regimen. Consider utilizing wellness applications or wearable gadgets to follow your work-out daily schedule, giving information on your exercises, pulse, and generally speaking action levels.

Track your rest designs by recording your sleep time, awaken time, and any disturbances during the evening. Note any progressions in your rest quality and how they correspond with your day to day propensities. Change your rest routine in view of this criticism, pursuing informed choices to streamline your rest.

Mental and Close to home Wellbeing Observing

Consistently survey your feelings of anxiety and the adequacy of your pressure the executives strategies. Keep a diary to record circumstances that cause pressure, your profound reactions, and the techniques you use to adapt. In the event that you find that specific stressors persevere, investigate extra survival techniques or look for help from an emotional wellness proficient.

Assess your capacity to appreciate people on a deeper level by pondering your correspondence and relational connections. Think about looking for input from confided in companions or partners to acquire understanding into regions for development. Keep on participating in exercises that advance profound prosperity and mindfulness, changing your methodology on a case by case basis.

Looking for Proficient Direction

Chasing after ideal wellbeing, make sure to proficient direction. Wellbeing and health experts, including nutritionists, fitness coaches, and psychological wellbeing experts, can give important experiences and backing custom-made to your particular requirements.

Nutritionist or Dietitian

In the event that you find it trying to explore the complexities of sustenance all alone, consider talking with a nutritionist or dietitian. These experts can survey your dietary propensities, give customized direction, and make a dinner plan that lines up with your wellbeing objectives. They can likewise address explicit dietary worries or limitations, it are met to guarantee that your nourishing necessities.

Fitness coach

A fitness coach can offer mastery in planning a viable and customized work-out daily practice. Whether you're a fledgling hoping to lay out an exercise routine daily practice or an accomplished individual looking to upgrade your wellness level, a fitness coach can give direction on legitimate structure, exercise force, and movement. They can likewise acquaint assortment into your exercises with keep you persuaded and locked in.

Psychological wellness Proficient

In the event that you experience difficulties connected with pressure, tension, or close to home prosperity, consider talking with a psychological wellness proficient. Analysts, advisors, and guides can offer restorative help, helping you investigate and resolve fundamental issues. They can likewise show methods for dealing with especially difficult times, stress the executives procedures, and methodologies for working on close to home versatility.

Keeping up with Long haul Achievement

The way to long haul progress in keeping a solid way of life lies in supportability and versatility. As you progress on your wellbeing process, be aware of the accompanying standards to guarantee all around was.

Consistency

Consistency is vital with regards to keeping a solid way of life. Laying out steady propensities in your eating regimen, work-out everyday practice, and rest designs supports positive way of behaving and adds to long haul achievement. Keep away from outrageous or impractical changes, selecting rather for continuous alterations that you can keep up with over the long run.

Adaptability

Life is dynamic, and unanticipated conditions might emerge. Embrace adaptability in your wellbeing intend to adjust to evolving circumstances. Assuming that startling difficulties impede your everyday practice, track down elective answers for keep focused. Being versatile permits you to explore snags without wrecking your advancement.

Reflection and Change

Routinely consider your wellbeing plan and survey its viability. Consider whether your objectives stay significant and practical, and be available to changing them in light of your developing necessities. Occasionally return to your activity intend to guarantee that it lines up with your ongoing way of life and yearnings.

Observe Accomplishments

Recognize and praise your accomplishments, regardless of how little. Perceiving your advancement builds up certain way of behaving and inspires you to forge ahead with your wellbeing process. Whether it's arriving at a wellness achievement, working on your dietary propensities, or effectively overseeing pressure, find opportunity to commend your achievements.

9.1 Summarizing key takeaways from the previous chapters

All through the former sections, we've investigated the complexities of making an extensive and customized wellbeing plan. The excursion started with a profound jump into the evaluation of your ongoing wellbeing status, incorporating a careful assessment of physical, mental, and close to home prosperity. By investigating your eating regimen, work-out daily practice, rest designs, feelings of anxiety, and survival techniques, you laid the basis for informed navigation and objective setting.

The significance of putting forth practical and feasible objectives arose as a urgent move toward the interaction. Whether zeroing in on actual wellbeing, mental prosperity, or close to home versatility, laying out clear targets gave guidance and inspiration. These objectives, going from dietary enhancements and work-out schedules to pressure the board methods and the capacity to understand people on a deeper level turn of events, filled in as the central focuses for making a customized activity plan.

The resulting sections dug into the quick and dirty of planning these activity plans, fitting them to individual requirements, inclinations, and ways of life. The actual wellbeing activity plan included continuous dietary changes, the joining of agreeable work-out schedules, and the foundation of solid rest propensities. On the psychological and profound front, care rehearses, stress the board procedures, and the ability to appreciate anyone on a deeper level upgrade became the dominant focal point. These way of life changes were created with an accentuation on reasonableness and manageability, guaranteeing they flawlessly coordinated into day to day existence.

Carrying out these way of life changes was featured as a vital part of the well-being venture. Responsibility and consistency were considered fundamental for progress, and a development outlook that saw difficulties as any open doors for learning was supported. The significance of celebrating little triumphs en route was underlined, cultivating a positive mentality and supporting the obligation to long haul prosperity.

Observing advancement filled in as a designated spot to check the viability of the individual wellbeing plan. Ordinary appraisals of dietary decisions, workout schedules, rest designs, feelings of anxiety, and close to home prosperity gave important bits of knowledge. Using instruments like food journals, wellness applications, and self-reflection, people could recognize areas of progress and change their arrangements as needs be.

The meaning of looking for proficient direction was highlighted as a way to improve the individual wellbeing venture. Nutritionists or dietitians offered mastery in exploring the intricacies of sustenance, fitness coaches gave customized exercise plans, and psychological well-being experts tended to pressure, nervousness, and close to home prosperity. These experts assumed urgent parts in supplementing individual endeavors and giving particular bits of knowledge.

Keeping up with long haul outcome in wellbeing and health was investigated through standards of consistency, adaptability, reflection, change, and the festival of accomplishments. Perceiving that life is dynamic, the requirement for flexibility and a receptiveness to adjusting wellbeing plans in light of changing conditions were considered basic. Reliable, reasonable propensities framed the establishment for enduring achievement, and the act of routinely thinking about and changing the arrangement guaranteed its continuous pertinence.

As we wrap up this thorough aide on making an individual wellbeing plan, it's critical to repeat the comprehensive idea of the methodology supported all through the sections. Wellbeing is certainly not a one-layered idea; rather, it includes physical, mental, and close to home prosperity. The combination of these components in a customized and noteworthy arrangement guarantees a fair and practical excursion toward ideal wellbeing.

All in all, your own wellbeing plan is a dynamic and developing guide, intelligent of your obligation to personal growth and prosperity. It's a demonstration of the comprehension that wellbeing is a deep rooted speculation, and every choice made in its interest adds to a more extravagant and seriously satisfying life. By consolidating the critical important points from these sections — self-evaluation, objective setting, customized activity plans, way of life changes, checking, looking for proficient direction, and keeping up with long haul standards — you set out on an extraordinary excursion toward a better and more energetic you. Keep in mind, the excursion is essentially as significant as the objective, and the little, steady advances you take today prepare for a better tomorrow.

9.2 Guiding readers in creating their personalized health plan

Setting out on the excursion of making a customized wellbeing plan is an extraordinary undertaking, promising superior actual prosperity as well as upgraded mental and profound strength. This thorough aide means to act as a compass, directing perusers through the mind boggling course of making a wellbeing plan that lines up with their one of a kind necessities, inclinations, and yearnings.

Surveying Your Ongoing Wellbeing Status

Prior to diving into the complexities of planning a customized wellbeing plan, considering your ongoing wellbeing status is basic. This includes a comprehensive assessment of your physical, mental, and close to home prosperity.

In the domain of actual wellbeing, examine your dietary propensities. What do your feasts comprise of, and how would they add to your general nourishment? Ponder the equilibrium of macronutrients, the consideration of fundamental nutrients and minerals, and the effect of your eating routine on your energy levels and safe framework.

At the same time, assess your work-out everyday practice. Observe the recurrence, power, and sort of proactive tasks you take part in consistently. Does your ongoing activity routine line up with your wellness objectives, advancing cardiovascular wellbeing, strength, and adaptability?

Past the physical, dive into your rest designs. Sufficient and quality rest is basic to generally prosperity. Consider your daily rest term, the nature of your rest climate, and any elements that may be influencing your rest.

Shift your concentration to mental and close to home wellbeing. Evaluate your feelings of anxiety and the survival strategies you utilize. What are the wellsprings of stress in your life, and how would you regularly answer them? Think about your close to home versatility and mindfulness, perceiving regions for development.

Putting forth Sensible and Reachable Objectives

Outfitted with an extensive comprehension of your ongoing wellbeing status, the subsequent stage is to laid out reasonable and reachable objectives. Objectives give an internal compass and inspiration, filling in as signals on your excursion to better wellbeing.

In the domain of actual wellbeing, lay out unambiguous targets for your eating routine. This could include integrating more products of the soil into your dinners, diminishing the admission of handled food sources, or guaranteeing satisfactory hydration. These objectives ought to be quantifiable and custom fitted to your singular inclinations and dietary requirements.

Going to work out, put forth reasonable wellness objectives that line up with your ongoing wellness level and wanted results. Whether it's rising the recurrence of your exercises, further developing perseverance, or dominating another actual work, pick objectives that challenge you without overpowering your ability.

For rest, lay out clear goals, for example, a predictable rest plan and a helpful sleep time schedule. Go for the gold number of long periods of rest every evening and execute unwinding procedures to upgrade the nature of your rest.

In the domain of mental and close to home wellbeing, put forth objectives connected with pressure the board. This could include integrating care rehearses, like reflection or profound breathing activities, into your everyday daily practice. Moreover, consider objectives for upgrading your capacity to understand individuals on a deeper level, for example, further developing relational abilities or looking for help from a specialist or instructor when required.

Planning Your Customized Activity Plan

With clear objectives set up, the following stage includes planning a customized activity plan that makes an interpretation of these yearnings into noteworthy stages. This plan ought to be adaptable, reasonable, and custom-made to your way of life, guaranteeing it's both possible and manageable.

Actual Wellbeing Activity Plan

Consolidate changes to your eating regimen slowly, zeroing in on little, feasible adjustments. Consider dinner preparing to guarantee better food decisions, steadily lessening the admission of sweet or handled food sources, and being aware of part estimates. If necessary, talk with a nutritionist for customized direction in view of your dietary inclinations and wellbeing objectives.

Plan a gym routine schedule that lines up with your way of life and inclinations. Pick exercises that you appreciate to improve the probability of consistency. Whether it's cardiovascular activity, strength preparing, or a mix of both, make active work a basic piece of your daily practice. Enroll the help of an exercise pal or consider employing a fitness coach for added inspiration and direction.

To work on your rest, lay out a sleep time schedule that signs to your body that now is the right time to slow down. Limit screen time before bed, establish a dull and calm rest climate, and hold back nothing rest plan. On the off chance that rest unsettling influences endure, talk with a rest expert to distinguish and resolve basic issues.

Mental and Close to home Wellbeing Activity Plan

Focus on pressure the board by integrating care rehearses into your regular routine. This could include brief breaks over the course of the day for profound breathing or care contemplation. Distinguish exercises that give you pleasure and unwinding, whether it's investing energy in nature, participating in a side interest, or interfacing with friends and family.

Improve your capacity to understand individuals on a deeper level through self-reflection and mindfulness works out. Journaling can be an important device for investigating your contemplations and feelings. Look for open doors for self-improvement, for example, going to studios or perusing writing that grows how you might interpret yourself as well as other people.

Carrying out Way of life Changes

Carrying out way of life changes requires responsibility and consistency. As you set out on your excursion to better wellbeing, be ready to experience difficulties and misfortunes. Embrace a development mentality that perspectives challenges as any open doors for learning and improvement.

Actual Wellbeing Way of life Changes

Integrate dietary changes step by step, trying different things with new recipes and tracking down better options in contrast to your number one food varieties. Consider signing up for a cooking class or investigating various foods to make the interaction charming. Remain aware of your dietary patterns, rehearsing instinctive eating to more readily comprehend your body's appetite and completion signs.

Focus on your work-out everyday practice by booking committed exercise meetings in your schedule. Make actual work a non-debatable piece of your everyday practice, and be adaptable in adjusting your exercises to oblige changes in your timetable. Celebrate little wellness achievements, whether it's finishing a difficult exercise or working on your presentation in a particular activity.

Develop sound rest propensities by making a loosening up sleep time schedule. Limit screen time before bed, establish a dull and calm rest climate, and hold back nothing rest plan. On the off chance that rest unsettling influences persevere, consider talking with a rest expert to distinguish and resolve fundamental issues.

Mental and Close to home Wellbeing Way of life Changes

Coordinate care rehearses into your everyday existence by integrating short reflection meetings or care practices into your daily schedule. Use care to explore unpleasant circumstances, zeroing in on the current second as opposed to becoming overpowered by future vulnerabilities. Develop a positive mentality by rehearsing appreciation and reexamining negative contemplations.

Support your capacity to appreciate people on a profound level by effectively paying attention to other people and trying to grasp alternate points of view. Participate in transparent correspondence, offering your viewpoints and sentiments in a valuable way. Focus on taking care of oneself exercises that give you pleasure and unwinding, whether it's investing energy with friends and family, participating in imaginative pursuits, or essentially going for a comfortable stroll.

Checking Progress and Changing Your Arrangement

Consistently screen your advancement to guarantee that your own wellbeing plan stays powerful and lined up with your objectives. Survey both quantitative and subjective parts of your prosperity to acquire a thorough comprehension of your general wellbeing.

Actual Wellbeing Checking

Keep a food journal to follow your dietary decisions and recognize examples or regions for development. Screen your energy levels, state of mind, and any actual changes as you make adjustments to your eating routine. Consider utilizing wellness applications or wearable gadgets to follow your work-out everyday practice, giving information on your exercises, pulse, and generally speaking action levels.

Track your rest designs by recording your sleep time, awaken time, and any interruptions during the evening. Note any progressions in your rest quality and how they relate with your everyday propensities. Change your rest routine in light of this criticism, going with informed choices to improve your rest.

Mental and Profound Wellbeing Observing

Consistently survey your feelings of anxiety and the viability of your pressure the board strategies. Keep a diary to record circumstances that cause pressure, your profound reactions, and the methodologies you use to adapt. In the event that you find that specific stressors continue, investigate extra strategies for dealing with especially difficult times or look for help from a psychological wellness proficient.

Assess your ability to understand individuals on a profound level by considering your correspondence and relational connections. Think about looking for input from confided in companions or associates to acquire understanding into regions for development. Keep on participating in exercises that advance profound prosperity and mindfulness, changing your methodology on a case by case basis.

Looking for Proficient Direction

Chasing after ideal wellbeing, go ahead and proficient direction. Wellbeing and health experts, including nutritionists, fitness coaches, and psychological wellbeing experts, can give important experiences and backing custom-made to your particular requirements.

Nutritionist or Dietitian

In the event that you find it trying to explore the complexities of nourishment all alone, consider talking with a nutritionist or dietitian. These experts can evaluate your dietary propensities, give customized direction, and make a feast plan that lines up with your wellbeing objectives. They can likewise address explicit dietary worries or limitations, it are met to guarantee that your healthful requirements.

Fitness coach

A fitness coach can offer mastery in planning a viable and customized work-out everyday practice. Whether you're a fledgling hoping to lay out an exercise routine daily schedule or an accomplished individual trying to upgrade your wellness level, a fitness coach can give direction on legitimate structure, exercise force, and movement. They can likewise acquaint assortment into your exercises with keep you propelled and locked in.

Psychological well-being Proficient

In the event that you experience difficulties connected with pressure, tension, or close to home prosperity, consider talking with an emotional well-being proficient. Clinicians, specialists, and advisors can offer restorative help, helping you investigate and resolve basic issues. They can likewise show methods for dealing with especially difficult times, stress the executives procedures, and methodologies for working on profound strength.

Keeping up with Long haul Achievement

The way to long haul progress in keeping a solid way of life lies in supportability and flexibility. As you progress on your wellbeing process, be aware of the accompanying standards to guarantee all around was.

Consistency

Consistency is vital with regards to keeping a sound way of life. Laying out steady propensities in your eating regimen, work-out daily schedule, and rest designs builds up certain way of behaving and adds to long haul achievement. Keep away from outrageous or impractical changes, selecting rather for progressive adjustments that you can keep up with over the long haul.

Adaptability

Life is dynamic, and unexpected conditions might emerge. Embrace adaptability in your wellbeing intend to adjust to evolving circumstances. In the event that unforeseen difficulties disrupt your daily schedule, track down elective answers for keep focused. Being versatile permits you to explore snags without wrecking your advancement.

Reflection and Change

Consistently think about your wellbeing plan and evaluate its adequacy. Consider whether your objectives stay pertinent and reasonable, and be available to changing them in view of your developing necessities. Occasionally return to your activity intend to guarantee that it lines up with your ongoing way of life and yearnings.

Observe Accomplishments

Recognize and commend your accomplishments, regardless of how little. Perceiving your advancement builds up certain way of behaving and spurs you to progress forward with your wellbeing process. Whether it's arriving at a wellness achievement, working on your dietary propensities, or effectively overseeing pressure, carve out opportunity to commend your achievements.

9.3 Encouraging ongoing self-reflection and adjustments to maintain a healthy lifestyle

Keeping a solid way of life is certainly not a static accomplishment yet a dynamic and progressing process that requires ceaseless self-reflection and changes. This pivotal part of the wellbeing venture guarantees that your own wellbeing plan stays pertinent, successful, and lined up with your developing requirements and desires. In this investigation, we dive into the significance of continuous self-reflection and give experiences into making changes that cultivate supported prosperity.

The Powerful Idea of Wellbeing

Wellbeing isn't an objective; it's a deep rooted venture set apart by turns, turns, and unforeseen diversions. Perceiving the powerful idea of wellbeing is basic to understanding the reason why continuous self-reflection and changes are fundamental parts of a manageable and successful individual wellbeing plan.

Life unfurls in unusual ways, and outer factors, for example, changes in work plans, relational peculiarities, or unanticipated moves can affect your capacity to stick to your wellbeing plan. Recognizing this reality permits you to move toward your wellbeing process with a feeling of flexibility, versatility, and a receptiveness to change.

Besides, individual wellbeing needs develop over the long run. As you age, experience new life stages, or stand up to various stressors, the prerequisites of your body and brain might move. What worked for you in the past may not be as powerful in the present. This understanding highlights the significance of routinely evaluating your wellbeing intend to guarantee it lines up with your ongoing conditions and objectives.

The Job of Self-Appearance in Wellbeing

Self-reflection is an incredible asset that enables you to acquire knowledge into your ways of behaving, propensities, and generally prosperity. It includes returning a stage to inspect your contemplations, sentiments, and activities, cultivating a more profound comprehension of yourself and your relationship with your wellbeing plan.

Ordinary self-reflection empowers you to:

Recognize Examples: By examining your ways of behaving and propensities, you can observe designs that might be impacting your wellbeing. Perceiving these examples permits you to settle on informed conclusions about whether they contribute decidedly or adversely to your prosperity.

Assess Progress: Considering your wellbeing process permits you to evaluate the headway you've made toward your objectives. Celebrate accomplishments, regardless of how little, and use misfortunes as any open doors for learning and development.

Grasp Triggers: Distinguish factors that trigger pressure, close to home eating, or interruptions to your work-out everyday practice. Understanding these triggers furnishes you with the information expected to foster successful survival techniques and systems to address difficulties.

Evaluate Close to home Prosperity: Self-reflection stretches out past actual wellbeing to incorporate profound prosperity. By investigating your profound scene, you can recognize regions that might require consideration, like stressors, tensions, or unsettled feelings.

Assess Inspiration: Evaluate your inspiration and obligation to your wellbeing plan. Understanding the basic reasons driving your quest for a solid way of life upgrades your capacity to remain persuaded and zeroed in on your objectives.

Down to earth Techniques for Self-Reflection

Integrating self-reflection into your routine doesn't need to be a complex or tedious cycle. Basic and down to earth techniques can be woven into your day to day existence to work with progressing contemplation and care.

Journaling: Keeping a wellbeing diary permits you to record your contemplations, sentiments, and perceptions connected with your wellbeing process. Note your day to day exercises, feasts, work-out schedules, and any difficulties or wins you experience. Over the long haul, checking on your diary gives significant bits of knowledge into examples and patterns.

Careful Minutes: Integrate careful minutes into your day. Whether through contemplation, profound breathing activities, or brief delays for reflection, these minutes encourage mindfulness and furnish a chance to check in with yourself.

Normal Registrations: Timetable customary registrations with yourself to evaluate your advancement and prosperity. These registrations can be week after week or month to month, offering assigned times for reflection on your objectives, difficulties, and changes required.

Input Circle: Look for criticism from confided in companions, relatives, or even wellbeing experts. Outer viewpoints can give important bits of knowledge into parts of your wellbeing that you might not have thought of.

Objective Reassessment: Intermittently rethink your objectives to guarantee they stay reasonable and lined up with your ongoing needs. Changes might be important in view of changes in your day to day existence conditions or wellbeing needs.

Changes as a Way to Development

Embracing the requirement for changes in your own wellbeing plan is definitely not an indication of disappointment yet an affirmation of development and mindfulness. Similarly as your life develops, so too should your way to deal with wellbeing. Consider changes as proactive measures that enable you to remain on a way of nonstop improvement.

Actual Wellbeing Changes

Dietary Changes: Your nourishing requirements might change over the long run because of elements, for example, age, movement level, or ailments. Intermittently evaluate your eating regimen to guarantee it lines up with your ongoing necessities. Consider counseling a nutritionist for customized guidance.

Adjusted Work-out Everyday practice: As wellness levels advance or life conditions change, your work-out routine might require change. Bring assortment into your exercises, change force, or investigate new exercises to keep your routine connecting with and successful.

Rest Streamlining: Changes in work plans, feelings of anxiety, or way of life might affect your rest designs. Change your rest normal on a case by case basis, trying different things with sleep time customs or changing your rest climate to improve the nature of your rest.

Mental and Close to home Wellbeing Changes

Stress The executives Methodologies: In the event that stressors in your life altering event, reevaluate your pressure the board techniques. Try different things with various procedures, like care, contemplation, or inventive outlets, to find moves toward that reverberate with your ongoing circumstance.

Profound Prosperity Practices: Investigate new practices to upgrade close to home prosperity. This could include consolidating exercises that give pleasure, cultivating significant associations, or looking for proficient help while confronting personal difficulties.

Correspondence and Limits: As connections develop, the requirement for compelling correspondence and limits becomes urgent. Change your way to deal with relational connections, guaranteeing that you focus on open correspondence and put down sound stopping points to safeguard your psychological and profound prosperity.

Exploring Difficulties with Flexibility

Difficulties are an unavoidable piece of any wellbeing venture. As opposed to review misfortunes as disappointments, think about them as any open doors for learning and versatility. At the point when mishaps happen, move toward them with a development outlook, understanding that difficulties give significant experiences into regions that might require further consideration or change.

Gaining from Difficulties: Think about the variables that added to the misfortune. Was it a transitory test, an adjustment of schedule, or a surprising stressor? Gaining from misfortunes assists you with recognizing expected sets off and foster systems to relieve their effect from now on.

Changing Objectives: Assuming difficulties uncover that specific objectives were excessively aggressive or ridiculous, consider changing them to more readily line up with your ongoing conditions. This might include setting more modest, more feasible achievements that add to long haul achievement.

Looking for Help: Go ahead and support from experts or friends and family during testing times. Whether it's a nutritionist, fitness coach, specialist, or a strong companion, having an organization of help can give important direction and support.

Developing Strength: Embrace mishaps as any open doors to develop flexibility. Strength is the capacity to return quickly from difficulties more grounded and more enabled. Every mishap is an opportunity to refine your systems, upgrade your methods for dealing with especially difficult times, and develop as a person.

Making a Culture of Persistent Improvement

The idea of progressing self-reflection and changes stretches out past the person to envelop the more extensive idea of making a culture of nonstop improvement. Similarly as organizations and associations flourish with versatility and development, so too might people at any point develop a mentality of constant improvement in their wellbeing process.

Embracing Deep rooted Learning: Move toward your wellbeing process with a mentality of long lasting learning. Remain inquisitive about new advancements in nourishment, wellness, and prosperity. This interest powers a proactive way to deal with your wellbeing, encouraging a feeling of strengthening and independence.

Adaptability as a Guiding principle: Develop adaptability as a basic belief in your wellbeing process. This includes not exclusively being adaptable in that frame of mind to dietary decisions, work-out schedules, and stress the executives yet additionally being versatile to the unavoidable changes that life brings.

Customary Wellbeing Check-Ups: Timetable standard wellbeing check-ups with medical services experts to screen key signs of your prosperity. These check-ups act as proactive measures, permitting you to recognize and address potential medical problems before they raise.

Local area and Shared Learning: Draw in with networks or care groups that share comparable wellbeing objectives. Shared learning and encounters inside a local area give extra viewpoints, bits of knowledge, and inspiration for ceaseless improvement.

The Groundbreaking Force of Reflection

Basically, progressing self-reflection and changes in your own wellbeing plan are not simply methodologies; they are extraordinary practices that lead to a more profound comprehension of yourself, your wellbeing, and your ability for development. By developing an outlook of consistent improvement and embracing the powerful idea of your wellbeing process, you position yourself on a way of supported prosperity.

www.ingramcontent.com/pod-product-compliance
Lightning Source LLC
LaVergne TN
LVHW011944070526
838202LV00054B/4794